The Silent Quarter
The Story of One

Viviane Lovato

The Silent Quarter: The Story of One

Viviane Lovato

Copyright© Year - MMXX

ISBN: 978-1-7364678-0-0 (Paperback Edition)
ISBN: 978-1-7364678-2-4 (Hardcover Edition)
ISBN: 978-1-7364678-1-7 (eBook Edition)

Cover Design by Sherwin Soy
Interior Design by Integrative Ink

What Readers Are Saying
About *The Silent Quarter*

"This book narrates Viviane's personal story, vividly bringing to life the challenges faced by every patient with Chronic Inflammatory Response Syndrome (CIRS); the harsh realities of living with CIRS; and direction for much-needed change. Interspersed with her story is well-referenced information about CIRS. Viviane's inner strength and determination provide hope, inspiration, and the message that there is light at the end of the tunnel. I plan to recommend this book to all my patients."

Dr. Ming Dooley – Certified Shoemaker Protocol Provider

"Captivating, heart wrenching, and informative!"

Layla El-Khoury – Biological Engineer, Choreographer and Dance Instructor

"*The Silent Quarter – The Story of One* sheds a clear light on the difficulties patients face when seeking acknowledgment and treatment for environmentally acquired illnesses (EAI), such as Chronic Inflammatory Response Syndrome (CIRS). The author's personal account highlights the need for education among the public and healthcare practitioners on these complex health conditions, as well as a the need for a paradigm shift to promote research that considers the impact of multiple hazard exposures from our environments over our lifetime. As an educator in environmental health sciences, I plan to recommend this book to my students as a primer for the next steps in understanding EAI."

Kelly A. Reynolds, PhD – Professor in Environmental Health Sciences, University of Arizona

"Informative, inspiring, and powerful. A *must* read for all who are debilitated by environmental conditions."

Lloyd Guérin – Founding board member of a spirituality center and Wisdom Elder

"Viviane Lovato takes you on her heart-wrenching journey thus far as a young woman grappling with devastating symptoms that are eventually identified as Chronic Inflammatory Response Syndrome (CIRS). This complex syndrome has forced many sufferers into 'medically-induced homelessness,' as they face health care providers who lack information about it and insurance companies who will not pay for the care needed. While the author acknowledges that this is not intended as a medical reference, it should be required reading for medical and nursing schools. For any health professional who has ever taken care of a patient with symptoms that cannot be explained, Viviane Lovato provides extraordinary insight into the patient experience and how a chronic debilitating illness such as CIRS can wreak havoc on a family – and how to find hope."

Dr. Jean Arlotti – Family Nurse Practitioner in Primary Care

"When you hear of people suffering from depression, anxiety, fibromyalgia, and chronic fatigue syndrome what comes to mind?

The Silent Quarter – The Story of One brings readers into Viviane Lovato's journey to uncover the cause of a debilitating illness robbing her of dreams of becoming a principal dancer at a well-respected ballet company. Her vivid descriptions of the "crashes" that confined her to her bed for months, along with her ability to find ways to persevere despite her illness is inspiring.

When tragedy or adversity hits, something beautiful is bound to emerge if you look for it. Through Viviane's courageous battle to find wellness, themes of amazing family support, self-advocacy, and GRIT are highlighted along an insightful education on an environmentally acquired illness with a genetic component called Chronic Inflammatory Response Syndrome (CIRS). And out of the Global COVID-19 Pandemic, this book emerged.

The diverse breadth of content in *The Silent Quarter – The Story of One* renders relevance and attraction amongst a broad group of readers. If you enjoy reading about families coming together to fight for one of their own and willing to sacrifice just about everything, this book is for you. If you are an environmentalist and like to dive deep into the medical consequences of poor air quality, this book is for you. If you are in the medical field and have patients with depression, anxiety, and chronic fatigue, this book is for you. Most importantly, if you are fighting to make your dreams happen despite setbacks and need the real-world perspective of someone that came close to giving up and found strength to overcome, Viviane's story is the perfect place to start."

Christy Quartlebaum, BSN, RN – Rare Disease
Access & Advocacy

Acknowledgments

Thank you to Mary Beshara, Margaret ("Peg") DiTulio, Dr. Ming Dooley, Dr. Linda ("Sunny") Goggin, Dr. Sandeep Gupta, Dr. Karen D. Johnson, Dr. Scott McMahon, Diane Parks, Kelly Reynolds, Michael Schrantz, Larry Schwartz, Dr. Jennifer Smith, and all the other professionals who participated in the interviews that made this book possible.

Special thanks to Dr. Scott McMahon for allowing me to use segments of our interviews in "A Word From Dr. McMahon" in order give the readers a glimpse into the gravity of what they are about to learn.

My deepest gratitude to all the donors who provided the funding to bring this book to a level of professionalism and beauty worthy of attention and praise. And thank you to my editor, Noémie Lovato, for helping me bring the tone, structure, and grammar in this book to a whole new level.

To Dr. Jean Arlotti, Dr. Ming Dooley, Layla El-Khoury, Lloyd Guérin, Christy Quartlebaum, Kelly Reynolds, and Michael Schrantz, thank you so much for taking the time to provide constructive and essential feedback on the book manuscript before finalization.

Thank you to Steve O'Connor for allowing me to use his beautiful photographs.

Thank you to my mentors, dance instructors, teachers, family, friends, acquaintances, and others who have believed in me and supported me throughout my life.

Lastly, I cannot express enough my gratitude toward my parents and brothers. They have been my constant companionship and support, without whom I would not have made it this far. No one could ask for a better family.

For my family,
who have been my constant and my rock,
and for all those whose lives
have been affected by
Chronic Inflammatory Response Syndrome (CIRS).

Table of Contents

A Word from Dr. Scott McMahon

During an interview with Dr. Scott McMahon, he talked to me about medically unexplained symptoms (MUS) and how Chronic Inflammatory Response Syndrome (CIRS) – a multi-system inflammatory illness brought on by a genetic susceptibility and exposure to environmental biological toxins – could be the key to understanding these symptoms that so many are experiencing. The reality and consequence of his words hit me, and I felt it important that, even before reading my story and learning what I have learned, people need to be aware of the gravity of the condition known as CIRS.

"...Additionally, there is another gap in understanding called medically unexplained symptoms (MUS). Fibromyalgia, functional abdominal pain syndrome, PMS [premenstrual syndrome], IBS [irritable bowel syndrome], chronic fatigue syndrome (CFS), TMJ [temporomandibular joint syndrome] etc. are typically considered MUS. That means they are symptoms or illnesses for which we have no pathophysiologic explanation and no biomarkers to tell if you really have the illness or not. These are some of the most common complaints in doctors' offices. Forty percent of all outpatient visits are for one or more MUS! The NIH [National Institute of Health], by itself, is spending $5.1 billion on researching just 6 of these symptoms this year [2020]. Literally, tens of millions of people in the U.S. suffer from one or more MUS! One expert in MUS published in 1999 that he felt all of these were probably variants of one single illness. I would agree, and it is CIRS. I say that for several reasons. Initially, I have been in medicine long enough to see definitions of various diagnoses change. When CFS was first discovered (1989 – Truckee High School, a WDB [water-damaged building]), it was a profound fatigue for unexplained reasons. Now it is a profound fatigue plus brain fog, sleep disturbances, muscle aches, weird neuro issues, stomach issues, innate immune abnormalities and more. Fibromyalgia in the late 80s was described as a profound muscle aching with sleep disturbances. Now, it is profound muscle aching with sleep disturbances plus brain fog, fatigue, weird neuro issues, stomach issues, innate immune abnormalities and more. See the overlap? I could say the same for MS [multiple sclerosis] and IBS. As their definitions change, they all look like CIRS. Indeed, when I see a person diagnosed with fibromyalgia, of <5 years origin, I usually see complete reversal of their fibro[myalgia] with CIRS treatment. Same for CFS, IBS etc. So my opinion is that the vast majority of these cases are unidentified CIRS, causing these MUS. CIRS has biomarkers and an explained pathophysiology, so it is not an MUS. Indeed, all of these MUS fall under CIRS – it is the explanation for most of these sufferers. If caught early, these people can be treated successfully and then subsequent MUS can be prevented. If caught late, they can be treated to some degree, but by then, secondary damage has probably occurred which we do not yet know how to fix completely.

So, while I cannot say how many [doctors] know about CIRS, I can say that most doctors see CIRS patients every day and many are unaware. I also know that doctors, NPs [nurse practitioners], PAs [physician assistants], NDs [doctors of naturopathy] etc. are discovering CIRS anew every day and my experience is that the numbers are mushrooming."

Introduction

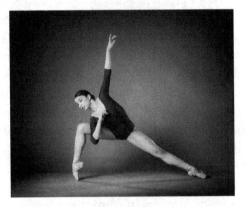

Viviane Lovato
Photo by Steve O'Connor (2016)

My name is Viviane Lovato. I am a 21-year-old Chronic Inflammatory Response Syndrome (CIRS) patient, aspiring professional ballet dancer, and CIRS advocate.[1] Though many people have told me I have a story to tell, I always thought I should wait until I've succeeded in more areas of my life to write a book. Who would want to hear of all the struggle when

---

1   I have experienced the health condition I am speaking about, I have talked to several experts in the field, and I have done much research on the subject. But I neither think I am, nor claim to be, an expert. I do cite my sources so that people may find more information, but this is not meant to be a scientific or academic book. To be clear, this book should not be relied upon as a substitute for professional consultation with a health care provider.

the ultimate victory, the "success", remains to be achieved? And how can I be vulnerable and paint the true image of myself with the knowledge that it is not yet well-developed?

However, recent events have made it clear to me that it is important that I share my story now, even if it isn't all tied up in a neat little bow as I would have liked.

CIRS has made my life more of a struggle than I ever expected, but this fight lends itself to an opportunity and a purpose. CIRS, a multi-system, multi-symptom inflammatory illness brought on by a genetic susceptibility and exposure to environmental biological toxins, is not a widely-known condition. Yet millions of people around the world are struggling with this illness, many of them misdiagnosed with other conditions. Even those who do know they have CIRS are faced with impossible barriers to the recovery of their health. The injustice – the incredible impossibility of so many people's situations, the devastating consequences of their inability to even begin treatment – boils my blood and breaks my heart. So many of these people's voices are stolen from them because their illness has consumed them. I, too, have been consumed by this illness. But I've been given a gift by those who've supported me. I now have my voice back. So I ask that you listen and walk with me as I recall my journey thus far and look forward with renewed hope and vigor into the future.

Chapter 1

The Beginning

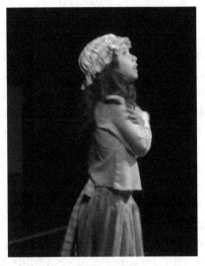

Viviane Lovato
Musical Theater Performance (2007)

When did the story of my struggle with Chronic Inflammatory Response Syndrome (CIRS) begin? Some might argue that, because CIRS is brought on by a genetic susceptibility, it started from the moment I was conceived. I certainly had to fight for my life from the beginning. If it weren't for the close watch of my mom's doctor, I would have likely been stillborn, due to a malfunction in how I received nutrients from my mother when I was in utero, a problem likely of a genetic origin. Similar genetic issues may also have played a role in

1

psychological and emotional issues I had starting around 6 years old. These issues continue to haunt me to this day; I carry with me a shame from these years, from the stories, and from the memories.

I remember a day in the first grade when I suddenly refused to go to school. I threw a fit, hiding under the table, creating quite a scene. These outbursts of anxiety and fear were not uncommon for me. And, eventually, they got to a point where, as a child who didn't even understand the concept of suicide, I was threatening it by standing out in the middle of the street. I was drawing dark scribbles and images, showing them to my mother, and saying, "This is how my stomach feels."

My parents did what most parents would do and brought me to a psychologist. Though the psychologist helped me to get a handle on these emotions, I continued to struggle with my emotional health throughout my childhood and adolescence. Eventually, I came to accept this as a part of who I am and labeled myself weak.

It is only recently that I've come to realize: I am anything but weak. Though I have no true closure on this time in my life, after hearing about PANDAS/PANS[2] – a condition common in children with the genetic susceptibility shared by CIRS that causes anxiety, obsessive-compulsive disorder (OCD), and other psychological symptoms – I felt a slight relief in that shame I've been carrying with me. I thought, "Perhaps there was a medical reason for those issues I had as a child; maybe I wasn't just a 'demon child' after all."

Besides this, in the early years, my childhood was pretty much what one would consider "normal". I was inspired by the arts, particularly by the performances of Audrey Hepburn, and I had a flair for entertaining others. So I started musical theater when I was around 7. But when I was 9, our situation was no

---

2   Pediatric Autoimmune Neuropsychiatric Disorder Associated with Streptococcal Infections/Pediatric Acute-onset Neuropsychiatric Syndrome

longer conducive to my continuing it, so my parents suggested I try ballet until we could resume musical theater. At first, being as stubborn as both my parents combined, I protested, disliking that I had to stop in the first place. But I came around to doing ballet as a means to an end. Little did I know... After my first *Nutcracker* performance with the ballet school, at 9 years old, I came off stage and told my mom, "That was the most fun thing I've ever done! This is what I want to do." It was the truth; and, for the next nine years, my life revolved around ballet.

Around the time I turned 11, my mom had her first relapse of mononucleosis. Over the course of a few years, she had periods of being bedridden, some days barely able to make it out of bed to use the bathroom. By the time I was 14, her illness had gotten so bad that I began to take care of her and take on a more adult role in the family. I looked after my brothers, who were 9 and 7 at the time. I prepared their lunches, helped them with school, and mediated their arguments. I helped my dad with the housework, like washing and cleaning. And, as my brothers got older, they joined in more, making their own meals and helping with chores.

Also around this time, I began to map out my plans for the future. I had decided, beyond a shadow of a doubt, that dance was what I wanted to do. After graduation from school, I would audition to join a company and start my career. I often daydreamed of the iconic moment that happened every year when a senior graduated from the dance school. At the end of the last performance of the season, the director would call them forward and tell the audience about them, maybe tell a funny story, and say with such pride what this dancer would go on to do. Some would go on to become physical therapists, others to dance with a company, others on to a prominent college to continue their education; but I was sure I'd be one of the ones going off to join a ballet company.

While these plans continued to form, silently and slowly my susceptibility to CIRS began causing issues in both my mental and physical health. But it was 2014 when my health issues became increasingly alarming. The frequent doctor visits and the lengthy search for answers began.

I thought I was a normal 15-year-old who struggled with normal teenage issues. I had just spent the last two summers training at prestigious ballet programs in Florida and Texas, and I was on my way to accomplishing my dreams. But despite being a highly motivated student, pre-professional dancer, and having everything to look forward to, I had a lot of trouble getting up in the morning. As it got more and more difficult to get out of bed in the morning, I employed the method of putting my alarm clock across the room to get myself moving in the morning. The result was a sprained wrist when my legs gave out instead. Every month, my menstrual cycles were coupled with cramping, fatigue, body aches, and migraines. But because my mom and the women in my dad's family all experienced similar cycles, I thought this was normal. In fact, I thought I had it good compared to other women in my family.

Toward the end of 2014, the fatigue and migraines that came with every cycle began to extend from one day of crippling fatigue, to two, to three. It began to get in the way of my studies and ballet, and it raised some red flags that maybe this was not normal. So my parents took me to the pediatrician. She examined me, tested a few things, and discovered only a vitamin D deficiency. Vitamin D deficiency can cause so many issues in the body, and it explained my symptoms, so I thought that must have been it. I got right on the vitamin D, eager to see the results. The doctor also recommended I see a neurologist for the migraines. He prescribed medication which, if I took it in time, helped manage the migraines.

But, despite the vitamin D treatment, the bouts of crushing fatigue and body aches continued to get worse, and more frequent, and last longer. By 2015, I was experiencing "crashes" where I would suddenly be too exhausted and in too much physical pain to attend dance classes or do my studies. I had a constant ringing in my ears for which the ENT (ear, nose, and throat doctor) could not pinpoint any cause. And the migraine medication eventually stopped working.

After seeing the pediatrician again, and finding nothing that could explain my fatigue, she suggested that I was just trying to do too much. So I dropped one of my more rigorous academic classes, and tried to focus most of my energy on being able to dance.

By the end of 2015, I was having regular migraines throughout the week and weekly crashes that mysteriously came on every Thursday. I'd barely make it through Wednesday's commitments, completely crash on Thursday, and if I was lucky, I'd recover enough by Saturday to do that day's class and rehearsals. Every week.

So per the doctor's recommendation, we added a sports nutritionist to the mix. Her finding was that I was just not taking in sufficient calories to support my physical activity and my hereditary fast metabolism. She told me to eat more overall, and to eat every two hours to head off the migraines. So I did just that. I always had a snack with me wherever I went, and I made sure to eat four hearty meals a day with snacks in between. I always ate in between class and rehearsal, to make sure I had enough "fuel" to dance and not crash by the end of the week.

It was working! Following the nutritionist's advice with obsessive consistency helped to hold the crashes and migraines at bay and brought their frequency back down to monthly.

Another rigorous summer training came around, this time in Kansas City, MO, and I made sure to tell them in advance about my dietary requirements since they would be providing meals. They were so supportive; they even gave me two of the boxed lunches every day. Despite the effort, I ended up becoming inexplicably ill with yet another crash toward the end of the intensive and had to sit out a few days to recover. As time passed, the crashes began to increase in length and, eventually, in frequency yet again.

By the end of 2016, these bouts of fatigue and pain would sometimes last an entire week. Still, I pushed forward with dance and school as though I would be fine.

When I looked back on doctors' notes and records to write this and get the timeline straight, I began to realize just how early on I began to get sick, and just how sick I was. Maybe I should have seen it at the time it was happening, but I think I was in such denial that I couldn't see the signs. I was refusing to recognize that something had gone terribly wrong in my body.

Then, in 2017, I had the worst crash yet.

Chapter 2

2017

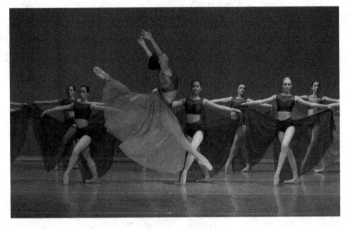

Viviane Lovato
Unkindest Year contemporary dance by Kristy Nilsson,
Photo by Julie Hacker (2016)

Starting in January 2017, my senior year of high school, I was primarily confined to my bed for three months. What had started as one of my week-long crashes dragged on into much much more. During this time, my body was barraged with full-on body pain, fatigue, insomnia, weakness, dizziness, neuropathy, migraines, and more. My mind was plagued by nightmares, depression, anxiety, OCD, and by the fear of the fact that I didn't know what was wrong with me – and neither did any of the doctors.

And my heart, well, this was one of the hardest times in my life. With the usual poor timing that life seems to be gifted in exploiting, I became alienated from my closest friend right before this crash hit. She was like a sister to me, but our friendship had become so fractured by that time that we were no longer each other's constant.

I did have one friend who visited me a few times in the seemingly endless three months. She brought me things to do and sat with me to keep me company. I had done the same for her when she was ill, and her return of this was something that further strengthened our bond and showed that she was a true friend. But she was the only one who ever came, and I can't recall many, if any, others who ever called or texted.

I was such a focused and driven young girl that friendships and relationships were not something I ever spent much time on. My focus was on my dancing and my studies. So apparently nobody else I went to school or trained with was close enough to me to reach out during this time and I, of course, did not reach out to them. I wasn't good at asking for help or comfort; I preferred to suffer through things by myself. Rarely would I reach out, even to my family, when I was suffering. By this time in my life, I never wanted anyone to see me weak, and it was difficult to appear strong when in so much pain. So my only consistent companionship during this time was my family. And in a turn of events, now my little brothers were caring for *me*. They brought me food, checked in on me from time to time, and tried to get me downstairs so I could be with them whenever possible, which in those three months was a rarity.

I have only a rough, bare-bones outline in my mind of this time, along with a few scary and vivid memories thrown in. I remember that, being home-schooled, my parents and I found ways for me to continue school and I graduated high school practically from bed, all while continuing the search for answers about my health. I remember that I did everything I could to be able to participate in the spring ballet performances. I remember that this was one of the most lonely, helpless, and hopeless times in my life. But, beyond that, I don't remember much. A lot of what I do share about this time has been a combination of reviewing medical notes, my family sharing their recollections with me, and sometimes my own recollections being triggered by those. I often wonder, is this lack of memory due to the brain fog I experienced? Do I simply not have these memories? Or is it a sort of PTSD, and I am unconsciously blocking out some very painful memories? I don't know, and I may never know.

However, because this was one of the pivotal times in my life and my journey, and because it exemplifies the suffering CIRS can cause, I feel the need to describe in more detail how this time impacted me and those closest to me. So I have included my family's recollections of this period. As difficult as it was, each of them agreed to share because they hope that one day it will make a difference for a family out there who's going through these very things.

Mom:
I wouldn't say I have vivid memories of this time period, either. Unfortunately, I was also struggling through my own diagnosis of ME/CFS [myalgic encephalitis/chronic fatigue syndrome], which included much of the same cognitive symptoms as Viviane, and lots and lots of ups and downs and push-crash cycles.[3] But my biggest feeling from this time is one of desperation as I tried to keep some semblance of normalcy in Viviane's life. Secretly, I was terrified that she would end up like me, and that we were both destined to be functionally dependent on others. But I refused to give up, and I was determined to help her keep going, pinpoint the cause, and get her better.

---

3 This is a reference to "push-crash syndrome" which is when patients who deal with exertion intolerance from chronic fatigue "push" through activities only to "crash" (experience severe fatigue and sometimes flu-like symptoms) afterward.

Leading up to this time, when each crash came on for her (at that time they were happening monthly and lasting 1-3 days), I remember having to regularly tell the Artistic Director that Viviane was "sick". How else do you say it? "Crashes" are what we had been calling my episodes of debilitating, or at times paralyzing, fatigue so it was already such a heavy and frightening word, and applying it to Viviane would have been an acceptance we weren't ready for. But eventually, as they got longer and more severe, there was no other word to describe them.

I remember the most jarring time I had to give that news, right at the start of when she was longest confined to her bed, when probably a week had transpired and she wasn't showing signs of recovery. I'm panicking inside, as a mom, not knowing what is wrong with my athletic child that she can't walk up and down the stairs without risking falling down them. And when I catch the director before class begins, I say, "Viviane has crashed again!"

Her response, in totality, was a slight pause and, "That's too bad."

The abruptness and finality of that just hit me. It was like what none of us had been wanting to admit was just affirmed: this was beyond a bump in the road that could be dealt with in the short-term, like a knee or foot injury. This was messy, and complicated, and completely disruptive.

Regardless, I went home and kept digging and digging for answers. Perhaps it was wrong of me, but that spring I allowed her to pour every ounce of her strength into her dancing, just trying to keep things feeling normal. After all, if she stopped dancing and spent all day in bed, how could I convince her that her fate was not the same as mine? Once she recovered enough to dance even a little bit, I remember days, getting home from rehearsals, when her dad had to carry her from the car to her bed, because her legs had nothing left and would give out – sometimes at the door, and sometimes before even getting out of the car.

On good days, in the morning she could come downstairs and do her school on the couch, where we could easily help bring her food and medicines. On bad days, she didn't leave her room until it was time to get dressed for ballet – if she could muster it – saving everything to get through a bit of class and whatever she could manage of rehearsal, by sheer willpower. I think dropping out of the shows entirely, for her, would have been like giving up and admitting the severity of the situation. I think it would have made it hopeless. And by March or April, we still thought recovery was just around the corner.

Dad:

In the beginning, Viviane's irritability and touchiness were minor, so I really didn't think much of it. I thought it was the teenage years, and that was it. But as things got worse, it started escalating to where we didn't have any communication because I was afraid that if I said something, she would take it a certain way and spiral into a melt-down. She was so touchy and fire-cracker like. So I just wouldn't talk to her. I would rather have no communication or little communication with my daughter than always start an argument or spark something that got her to a point where it was a longer, more frustrating conversation, or an explosion.

We didn't know what was going on. And I knew that ballet was her passion. I was proud to some extent, but to me, ballet was more of a curse than a gift. She was always in pain, always fatigued, always touchy. She gave everything to dance and school. So she had nothing left for anybody. There was nothing left for me or her mom or the family; it was just – that was it.

The other thing that stemmed from this was her loneliness. It was almost like a willing loneliness. It wasn't because she wanted it that way, but because her body wasn't able to give anything else to life or to others when she had spent it all on dance. It wasn't just family, but also friends or going out. She just didn't have anything left. At the time, it was like a loneliness that she *didn't know she was putting herself through because it was a result of her body being unable to keep up with everything.*

And I remember how much I just wanted to give her a hug, but I couldn't, because I was afraid I'd physically hurt her.

Little Brother:

Before CIRS affected Viviane so much, she would make up stories and play make-believe and other games with us.

Things changed during high-school/college. I remember her telling us not to even talk to her in the mornings, otherwise she would lose it. [Mornings were so difficult for Viviane that she couldn't even manage conversation. But the boys, excited that she was up, would quickly go and tell her what exciting thing they had been doing that morning.]

During the times she was really sick, I wouldn't see her for the majority of the day, because she was in bed in her room.

I also remember that she would always, without fail, ask us if we had washed our hands before making her food, or even bringing it upstairs. If we didn't, she would freak out, so we all agreed to just lie to her if we had forgotten. [This was due to Viviane's OCD being so heightened during this time. Upon learning of this in the course of writing this book, Viviane told him, "You did the right thing."]

Youngest Brother:

I remember bringing Viviane food every morning, sometimes lunch and dinner as well. Basically bringing all her meals. I also remember having to fill up her little water cup what felt like every few seconds. That was pretty much it. That was just life. Someone was always sick. Mom got sick starting when I was around 6. So either Mom or Viviane was sick and, by that point, it was just normal. I knew that it wasn't completely normal, but I knew that it was my normal. So I didn't think much about it.

The impact this time had on my family and on me has been strong and lasting. Even after just three months of being primarily confined to my bedroom and bed, I developed a dislike, and perhaps what could be considered a minor phobia, of bedrooms. Even now, I refuse to sleep in a bedroom, instead sleeping on a futon in the living room. And, as I look back on this time to write this book and read my family's memories, I still get that horrible feeling of fear and painful recollection in my gut and chest.

But there have also been positive impacts, even from something as challenging and harsh as this. My family and I have strong relationships and bonds with one another because of all we've been through together – this time included. I developed a powerful gratefulness toward the simple things in life. Going for a walk, feeling the sun's warmth grace my face, standing at the sink and washing the dishes, folding clothes. Things like this, even things I once found tedious and annoying, are so much more enjoyable now that I know what it is like to be unable to do them.

Chapter 3

Doctor, Doctor

*"Desperation is a necessary ingredient
to learning, or creating anything. Period."*
- Jim Carrey

During this crash, several specialists and doctors assessed
and treated me. The new family medicine doctor we
were seeing treated me again for a vitamin D deficiency. My
acupuncturist did what he could, and once sent me back to
the family medicine doctor after detecting irregularities in my
pulse but, by the time we got in to see the doctor, the episode
had subsided. Then at one point in late February, for days I felt
I could not breathe and my chest felt like it was caving in on
me. Every time I sat up or got up, I felt dizzy. Heightening to
a scary point late one night, and having no answers up to this
point, I ended up going to the ER. The ER doctors couldn't find
anything wrong with me, so they referred me to a cardiologist
and an endocrinologist.

The cardiologist, who seemed rather disinterested and
dismissive of my case – taking a phone call mid-appointment
without explanation or apology – found only that my blood
pressure was quite low and recommended I take salt pills or
eat salt when I experienced shortness of breath and dizziness.
So salt became my go-to. I'd pop some in my mouth and feel
a slight decrease in the dizziness and shortness of breath for a

few minutes. It worked to some extent, so I supposed my low blood pressure was to blame. Who cared why, right? I talked to a doctor, and he gave me the usual band-aid solution.

The endocrinologist found some significant hormonal abnormalities and hypothyroidism, and also discovered I was experiencing peripheral neuropathy.[4] He seemed sure these hormonal abnormalities were what was causing my problems, and I was put on medication to treat it. I was hesitant to believe that we had found the cause and had a solution. But one visit, a well-meaning nurse said, "Don't worry, honey. Once he's done with you, you're going to feel like a new person!"

At this point, I was beginning to develop a cynicism toward these over-confident statements that, each time, brought hope. But they still affected me, and I desperately wanted to believe them. And, regardless of what I believed, I followed the instructions religiously.

In March of 2017, while I was seeing the endocrinologist, I went to see an internist that specializes in chronic fatiguing illnesses. This internist knew what she was talking about, and she was constantly reading the latest and greatest research in her field. Her office had what seemed like millions of books. I was diagnosed with chronic fatigue, fibromyalgia, secondary dysautonomia, and two significant MTHFR mutations[5], and she explained how and why each of these things was affecting me. My methylation deficiencies and my high activity levels, along with some unknown initiating cause, had depleted my glutathione and ATP levels. According to this diagnosis, all we had to do was raise those things in my body, and it would take over, and things would go back to normal.

---

4 Peripheral neuropathy is weakness, numbness, and pain, usually in one's extremities, as a result of damaged nerves.

5 MTHFR mutations are mutations in the methylation process, which our bodies use to produce energy in the form of ATP, among several other things.

I was afraid to hope, but it all made sense. So I dared to hope, just a little. The internist put me on high doses of methylfolate for the methylation deficiencies, as well as weekly infusions of glutathione and ATP for the fatigue, fibromyalgia, and dysautonomia. As with all the other regimens and treatment plans that came before, I followed her instructions and advice to the letter, my OCD finding a useful place in keeping me on track.

At this point in time, I couldn't yet differentiate between what I like to call "chemical emotions" – emotions brought on by chemical imbalances – and emotions that came from what I was feeling about my life or things that happened. This became dangerously problematic when the methylation supplement the internist put me on brought on the worst depressive episode I have experienced to this day. Over the years, I had many depressive episodes as a kid and fantasized about suicide more than once as an adolescent. This time I came closer to taking my life than I ever had before. The thing about these "chemical emotions" is they create a vicious cycle where the "chemical emotions" and "natural emotions" feed off one another, amplifying, and continuously building to a point that neither would have reached on their own.

I remember lying on the floor crying, feeling such emotional pain and hopelessness. For so long I had been hating the pain, the weakness, and the dependency I lived in every day. I felt like I was a burden to my family. I was constantly sick and they were constantly caring for me. A voice in my mind said to me, "They would be better off without you." I had heard this in my mind before but never so clear, and it never felt so true. I remember fighting it, thinking how taking my life would be the wrong choice and that I didn't really want to die. But that voice pushed on saying, "Don't be selfish. They are spending so much money, time, stress, and energy on you. They deserve better. Do it." I looked up to see the bottle of pain killers I kept in my room for when the fibromyalgia got too bad. I reached up and grabbed it. I got as far as opening the bottle, when I could feel the part of me that knew this wasn't right crying out, "Something is wrong, something is really wrong. This isn't right." I reached for the phone, thinking I just needed to get someone on the phone before I did something irreversible. I called but there was no answer. I panicked and went back to my thoughts. They urged me to just end it all and save my family from further suffering because of me. But they also urged me to try to call someone else, to just try, to just reach out. Finally, the thoughts that voiced doubt that taking my life was really the best course of action became strong enough to cause me to reach for the phone once more and this time call my mom. I remember feeling so guilty for calling the very person who I thought my suicide would have saved and helped. "How selfish of you," I remember hearing in my mind as the phone rang. She answered, and I don't recall what I said or what transpired. I just remember her coming upstairs, picking me up in her arms, and holding me. I remember her freaking out, worried, angry, alarmed, frightened…

After this, I only remember that, eventually, the methyfolate supplement seemed to pass through my system and it was as though I was a different person. I looked back on what had just transpired and it felt like it had happened to someone else. I remember thinking, "What in the world? Was that really me? I can't believe that was me. I know my parents would be hurt worse by my death than by my living like this. I know killing myself wouldn't help anyone. And I know I don't want to die. What the f--- was that?" It was one of the most frightening and strange experiences of my life. I remember a sense of relief that I hadn't killed myself, and I'm so grateful that some piece of me was able to peek through the storm of "chemical emotions" and reach out for help.

As difficult as it is to share things like this, I want people to know that they are not alone. That, when something like this happens, it doesn't make you weak or less, and there is no reason not to reach out for help, <u>ever</u>. I also want all those who are struggling with illness and feel they are a burden on their loved ones to know: despite what you may hear from your own mind or even from the mouths of others, the world needs you. You are completely unique; no one else can do what you can and will do in this life and in this world. Remember that.

To get help or to talk to someone at any time – day or night – those in the US can reach out to the National Suicide Prevention Lifeline: 1-800-273-8255

≡

After being treated by the internist and the endocrinologist for a short time, I could finally be up and about on some days. Just having "good days" and being up and out of bed was a significant improvement to me. I was on the right track, moving forward finally. So I eagerly threw myself back into ballet. I had to withdraw from half of the performance pieces, as I could still only manage part of class and rehearsals. The rest of my time was spent at home lying down and doing school, and most of the time I still needed help getting food, taking care of myself, and getting up the stairs, especially when I had spent all of my energy trying to get through dance. But I needed to dance. The suffering I felt was only magnified by the fact that I was unable to dance, so I was so happy to be able to go back, even if it was in the smallest amount. It was my top priority. I sacrificed everything – family time, socializing, school, anything and everything that I had to – just to dance for a few hours a week and not have to drop out of all of the performances for the spring.

I pushed through more pain and fatigue than I care to remember. I remember I would "rest" all day at home, lying in bed, or sitting on the couch, saving all my energy and pain tolerance for dance. It was my only relief – my only escape from the uncertainty, fear, loneliness, and denial that plagued my mind and soul. So I pushed through classes and rehearsals. I'd be meticulous in rationing what little energy I had throughout the day to put it all into dance.

I would do everything the doctors said to try to get even just a little more energy to get through a show. I packed and ate the snacks the sports nutritionist had recommended. I sucked on the salt the cardiologist recommended. I took the medicine my endocrinologist prescribed. And I went in weekly for the infusions my internist recommended. I'd even get an extra infusion right before a run of shows.

During performances, I'd go on stage and, for a few minutes, the audience and I were the only things that existed. What I was giving them out on that stage was all that mattered. For a few blissful moments, I would forget the pain, the fatigue, the fear, and become lost in the performance. But the second I got off stage, everything came crashing back. I would quickly find a place to collapse where I would not be in the way or get run over. I'd take my medicine, eat my food, suck on some salt, lie down, and await the next time my role required me on stage. This was my senior year of high school and of dance.

My plans for after high school had been clear cut since I was 14 years old. That spring, I was to audition for ballet companies I had researched and selected throughout the years leading up to this point. I even had an option to revisit possible employment with a company that had offered me a position in 2016. I refused to give up hope on this vision. In January, right before the big crash, I had pushed myself through an audition and got accepted to a summer program with a company that I wanted to dance with professionally, where I was hopeful to be considered for a year-long traineeship.

But as summer was approaching, I was running out of time to heal. I was having some better days, but I still couldn't get through three hours a day of training, not to mention have anything left over to take care of myself. It was clear: I had to inform the company that I would not be able to attend their program that summer. This was one of the hardest moments during this time in my life. Up until that point, I had refused to believe that the plan I had since I was 14 years old had suddenly and completely fallen apart. I had fought to make it work with at least some resemblance to my original plan. Though I still believed this would just be a small delay, the truth was that it was just the beginning, and my plans for the future were more uncertain than they had ever been.

Chapter 4
Up and Down Again

"Fight. Anyone can do it when it feels good.
When you're hurting, that's when it makes a difference,
so you have to keep fighting."
- Erin Cafaro

Through the second half of 2017, my health progressed to some extent; however, that progress was not only insufficient, but it also began to fade. As the year went on, I pushed through more and more fatigue and more and more pain. So as we continued to work with the internist, we added a different kind of medicine and a new approach. In January of 2018, we went to a chiropractor/nutritionist. My cynicism was at an all-time high, but this new doctor was so sure that he could find the piece that the internist was missing, and his staff wasn't shy in sharing with me all the success stories of his previous patients. If I had the energy to, I'd force a slight smile and nod, feigning belief in their words and promises. This new doctor said my body was unable to break down and get nutrients from food, and he had several ideas to help with this. Like so many before him, he was confident that he'd have me better in no time and that his treatment would be the breakthrough for my health. Each doctor seemed to be trying to give me hope by making promises of recovery, not realizing that in doing this, they were doing me a disservice because they could not fulfill those promises. After following his advice, once again obsessively though with less enthusiasm than before, I saw results in some of my symptoms. The migraines and stomach pain responded well to the treatment, but nothing was moving the needle on everything else.

I continued to push through dance through the spring of 2018 and took on a light college load. And by "light", I mean one course. At times I was able to do some dance and take care of myself at home, but my condition was very unstable. There were times when I would barely make it through dance or didn't make it to dance at all, and I needed help with everything. Then there were times when I could dance and still sit up with my family to play a game at home. To be honest, I don't remember many of the details from this time either. As before, I don't know if my lack of memory is just part of my condition or my brain's attempt to block out some very painful moments. My mom, however, kept a detailed record of how I felt throughout this time, watching for patterns or improvements. As I read through this record years later, I came to realize that this was a great documentation of what I went through in 2018. I've included some of it here with additional notes of my own of select memories that I do have of this time and of memories that were triggered when reading through these notes.

Notes on V [Viviane] (2018)

2/6/18 Tuesday – V felt increasingly bad, much like she was when on allergy shots. Was not able to finish her dinner. Too tired.

Note from V: I do remember those allergy shots. After taking them in November 2017, I would feel the worst fibromyalgia pain I've ever felt. By this point in time, I rarely cried for pain, but this pain brought me to tears. All that I could feel was the pain. My entire body was on fire with it, throbbing, and just the clothes against my skin were a source of utter torture.

I would have given anything to make the pain go away. I took some pain killers despite the knowledge that it could set back the healing of my fragile stomach. But I found minimal relief with the pain killers and stopped the shots. But now something else was causing a similar effect.

2/7/18 Wednesday – V was not able to come down for breakfast. Ate in bed. Said everything hurts, even sometimes breathing. Soon after, stopped taking liver cleanse [supplement]. Recovered back to baseline in 36hrs.

2/14/18 Appt. with internist. Began allergy injections with diluted vials. Also appt. with chiropractor/nutritionist. Began IPS [L-Glutamine and other compounds for gut healing].

Note from V: Yeah, we tried those shots again. The idea was that maybe it was my allergies that were causing all of the fatigue, pain, and stress on my body. So we reasoned that we had to fix the allergy issues for me to get better. I really did not want to, but I was desperate for progress and rationalized with myself that the diluted vials would be better, just as the doctor assured me.

2/19/18 Today she fixed food, washed two loads of laundry, prepared her meds for the week, studied for a test, and danced normal percentage (40-50%). Also administered 2nd allergy shot.

Note from V: The director and instructors at the dance school wanted me to keep dancing as well, so from the time I got sick for as long as I needed, they were flexible in allowing me to do as little as necessary as I healed. They also knew that I would put dance above all else and knew I would be responsible, making sure to meet the obligations required to be a part of performances. And that's exactly what I did.

2/20/18 Not feeling well by afternoon. Woozy, dizzy, legs hurt, tired.

2/25/18 Sunday – spent day sewing [pointe] shoes, fixed breakfast and lunch by herself, and did a few more things around house. Caught herself humming while walking! (Did not do shots as scheduled on Thursday 2/22)

Note from V: The allergy shots' negative impact on my body was just plain excruciating and unmanageable, so I decided not to do them anymore, even diluted.

3/18/18 Finishing week of spring break. Not dancing but doing more around house. Preparing her own meds and vast majority of her food. Doing school and self-portrait assignment. Personality and actions more characteristic from when she was healthy.

3/24/18 Saturday after first week after spring break. V has had the best week in over a year. She danced very hard on Tuesday and felt pain after but was able to do almost all of 1 hr modern [class] on Wednesday, and still did part of class and rehearsal on Thursday. By Thursday night, she said she was tired but didn't feel 'dead' and wasn't desperate for a rest day. Today she did 45min of class, all 5 variations of [Twisted] Tangos in a row plus some 2nd runs, then ran Polonaise and cleaned variation for Sleeping Beauty.

3/29/18 Thursday – Despite being [menstrual] cycle week, V is having a second strong week in a row. She is consistently making her food, including salads, and juice, as well as school. Dysautonomia has been minimal, still no migraines, and stomach pain and nausea are still absent. Has done about 45 min of class and rehearsals as needed without sitting out of her roles.

5/9/18 Wednesday – After having a third solid week, V's symptoms returned. She began to have more dysautonomia and getting through spring show April 21 & 22 was quite tough. After shows, she decided to pull out of all recital pieces except modern, so she has been skipping all classes except modern and only running her own rehearsals [for her choreography piece] twice a week. Throughout, her body still had the fibromyalgia, though dysautonomia was not as bad as before. In the last week or so, her stomach has been increasingly more painful after meals such that she has lost all appetite even more than usual and she is eating a lot less. It doesn't hurt after eating salads or vegetable juice, but any protein or fat meals cause considerable pain. Last night she called me at 1am afraid because she got such a strong pang, even though she last ate at 7:30 and only had vegetable juice at 9ish.

Note from V: As you may have noted, there was a lot of up and down during this time. This was extremely difficult because every rise and fall held the all too familiar hope and disappointment. I would try my best to reserve any excitement, but so many times I dared to hope just a little that maybe it would last, only to be crushed again, and again, and again. Also, I think the ups and downs of it all contributed to how those around me perceived me. It was confusing how I could dance as much as I did and then suddenly be so sick that I had to severely minimize what I was doing or sit out. What condition would cause something like that? Still, all things considered, there was minimal judgment, and I believe this is because of a dancer who came before me. She had postural orthostatic tachycardia syndrome (POTS), a type of autonomic nervous system disorder (or dysautonomia) that manifests in a similar fashion to CIRS. The school staff had experienced what it was like for her, with her ups and downs, so they had that previous experience to draw from to be supportive and to accommodate me. The fact that the majority of the instructors were empathetic and kind also contributed to the level of support I received. I can only hope that if someone else comes along who has a similar condition, I was able to give them the same gift the dancer with POTS gave me, and make it even just a little bit easier on them. Because, when dealing with something like this, no one should have to face judgment as well.

6/10/18 Sunday – Upon reading more about celiac disease [due to her brother being diagnosed as likely celiac and both of them having the gene for it], I learned that many, many of Viviane's symptoms are consistent with celiac or non-celiac gluten sensitivity. Decided to test her for celiac in the best way we can without having insurance. In run up to [antibody] test I made sure she was still eating gluten. She began eating a little more than her usual. Her symptoms that manifested over the week included: stomach pain, bloating, increased constipation, increased peripheral neuropathy, severely heightened fibromyalgia pain (cannot be touched), and two oral canker sores. Blood test is tomorrow, so she will only eat minimal gluten today, then decided she will remove it. Will monitor her ability to exercise over the next few months after elimination of gluten.

Note from V: I remember the gluten test. That was horrific. I upped my intake of gluten in preparation for the test, and the result was all different kinds of pain increased in all areas of my body. Though I was never diagnosed with celiac, I am clearly, at the very least, gluten intolerant. Even cross-contamination has an impact on my body, and I must keep the kitchen completely gluten free and be very careful when going out to eat. Although I did much better off of gluten than on it, it did not turn out to be the one thing that was holding me back from health as we had hoped.

6/13/18 Wednesday – Still feeling absolutely horrible. Fibromyalgia (still hurts to be touched), fatigue, psychological symptoms, mood swings, constipation, urination frequency/

urgency. Got a third canker sore. [Celiac test came back inconclusive. Ordered more tests to get more information.]

6/17/18 Sunday – Last night the fog began to lift – V's sense of humor began to show and she began to have social conversation. She mentioned noticing the difference in brain chemistry, noting that her thoughts were more logical and typical of where she is, not hitting the rails as she often used to do. She even sat with us to watch a movie at night. Still could not be touched or hugged. Today she came down[stairs] and helped with her breakfast and other meals. And for the first time since she went down [crashed], she ate dinner downstairs at the table. Also had a conversation with Pépère [grandfather] and went to take her Epsom salt bath after he left. Today the fog was definitely lifted, as her personality was back.

Note from V: The gluten antibody tests came back negative. A later endoscopy showed some flattening of my villi, but the doctor couldn't conclusively say whether that was from gluten or from a medication I was on.

6/18/18 Monday – V's personality is definitely back. She is also moving a little faster through the house and up and down the stairs. Doesn't look as weak anymore. Still painful to touch. Had prelim consult with doctor in CA. Will have appt. tomorrow. Would like her to come for appt. as she said her case is complicated. Due to no job [her dad was unemployed at the time], they will get some tests first. More info on that to come. [We ended up not going any further with the doctor in California.]

6/20/18 Wednesday – V went downhill this afternoon. Started her period yesterday. Feeling woozy, visual disturbances.

Five days later, I found myself visiting yet another doctor. A new kind of doctor who would take an approach that none before her had taken.

Chapter 5
The Spark

*"If you are willing to do whatever it takes for
as long as it takes, success is just a matter of time."*
- Ruben Gonzalez

At the end of the 2018 spring season, one thing became clear to me: If I continued to push through the pain and the fatigue, my love for ballet would be at risk. Pliés, tendus – those simplest of ballet moves – caused pain to reverberate throughout my body, starting with the pins and needles feeling of neuropathy in my feet every time my foot moved against the floor. Nearly every day for 1½ years, I danced through this pain. During performances, the adrenaline made me forget – the pain, the uncertainty, the ever-present effort of denial, and the fear – for a few blissful moments. But most of the time I was dancing, I was in pain. And then, when I would come home from dancing, the pain would hit even harder. So naturally, my mind had begun to associate ballet with pain. I came to realize the sad truth: that association would only lead to my mind eventually convincing me that my passion and career is too painful to continue. That constant pain was beginning to smother my love of dance. I could not see a path forward for dancing professionally other than the one I was on, but I also realized that if I kept doing what I was doing, eventually I would not even desire a path forward. I couldn't let that happen. It was the voices and faces of those who came up to me after performances in tears because they were so touched; the faces of the young girls who were inspired by me; the beautiful necklace that one of these girls gave to me because she enjoyed watching me dance so much; or the gift left for me after a show of *The Nutcracker* by a complete stranger who said I was "the best Snow Queen" she had ever seen, teaching me that I have something unique to offer, something that, to her, set me apart. I wanted to be able to explore all of this. I wanted to explore using my art to impact and inspire people, and I wanted to discover what my unique artistry really is and could be. All these things echoed in my mind, heart, and soul. I knew I couldn't risk destroying something that not only gave me so much joy, but also gave other people this much joy and inspiration. So for the sake of my passion and my art, I stopped dancing in May 2018. I was determined that this would be temporary. That I would come back to dance without pain, and be able to love and enjoy it once more without that fog of agony over it.

I just didn't know how.

≡

By the summer of 2018, I had been following the treatment protocols of the internist and the endocrinologist for a year, and the nutritionist/chiropractor for half a year. I focused on resting and staying in shape as much as I could without pushing myself too hard. I swam from time to time, did some easy exercises when I could, stretched, and read motivational and self-help books to try to keep a positive mindset. In July, I managed to attend a choreographer's training project in Kansas City, MO, as a choreographer, so I wouldn't be required to dance but could at least do something to progress my career and gain some new knowledge. All of this while my parents and I continued in our search for answers, as we had been doing for nearly three years.

I was still under the care of the internist and the chiropractor/nutritionist, but my belief in either one's ability to get me healthy was waning. And I was tired of it all. I remember a moment in the car with my mother after an appointment with the chiropractor/nutritionist. He had just given us new recommendations for a new treatment plan. But we had both lost faith in him. I had lost faith in all doctors. I had given up hope that any doctor could fix me.

And I was tired. So tired. It was a horrible roller coaster ride of hope, crush, hope, crush, hope, crush. I couldn't take any more. I was just done.

≡

Back in 2017, when I was at my lowest low, my dad had handed me a book called *The Courage to Succeed* by Ruben Gonzalez. I vividly remember the moment. I was curled up on the floor, feeling hopeless and powerless, when my dad walked in and said, "You might want to read this; it's from a good friend of mine." He placed the book in front of me and left without another word. It took some time but, eventually, I read this book and later on another one of Ruben's books. At some point, one of those books led me to create a card with my main goals written on it and read it every morning and every night for months. On the front it read:

*"I am a ballerina/principal dancer at a professional
and well-respected ballet company."*

On the back it said:

*"I am ballerina/principal dancer because:
I take care of my body,
I workout/dance Monday-Saturday,
I <u>love</u> dancing,*

and I am willing to do whatever it takes
for as long as it takes."

My "workout" at the time was non-existent. Either I did gentle stretching with about four pelvic tilts and maybe some toe lifts for my bunions, or nothing at all. So many days I skipped reading that line and just focused on the others. Reading this consistently somehow programmed my mind to believe that I would make it to my dreams no matter what. I believed I would dance again, but I did not believe I would ever be healthy again. So I pushed away all thoughts that would creep to my mind like: *How can I get where I want to go like this? How can I even live like this?* I just went from day to day doing whatever I could and knew to do, without a thought to the future. I just knew I had to dance again, no matter what.

My mother, seeing things clearer than I was, had simply lost confidence in the doctors we had already seen. Each doctor provided a piece of information from their own specialty and perspective. The pediatricians had found some basic vitamin deficiencies. The sports nutritionist recognized that my body needed more food. The endocrinologist had diagnosed the hormonal irregularities. The internist found some methylation deficiencies and saw my body's struggle to produce energy. But no one had put it all together and answered the question *why*. My mom was determined to find someone who could take a more comprehensive approach, and find the underlying cause that was wreaking havoc on my body.

In mid-June, following months of ups and downs without any major progress, my mom learned about functional medicine practitioners and found one about 45 minutes away that came very well recommended. She was a pediatrician who also went back to train in functional medicine. My mom talked to me about this new doctor, and how she thought we should let her take a look at me. But I told her I was done – that I didn't want to go through another doctor, and all that comes with them. She listened and understood, but she refused to let me give up. So I went into that appointment without any hope, without any belief that this doctor could do anything to help me that the others hadn't already tried. And the only reason I went, is because my mom made me.

Before the first appointment on June 25, 2018, the doctor gathered an extensive medical history; she asked questions concerning things as far back as when my mom was pregnant with me. The medical history form was several pages long and very detailed. The week before the appointment, I had even more questionnaires to complete, as well as something called a Visual Contrast Sensitivity (VCS) test to complete (which I failed).[6] At our first appointment, she walked us through all the significant points of all the information I had submitted and she had analyzed. She said, "You may have Chronic Inflammatory Response Syndrome, and I really think this could be what's keeping you down." I remember distinctly that she made no promises that this was the answer, or that this was the end-all, be-all. She simply said that this is what she *thinks* is causing many of my symptoms. She tested me further for that but also ran more tests to find out what other health issues and conditions may have been affecting my body. She also explained to me in detail what CIRS is.

"Chronic inflammatory response syndromes (CIRS) are multi-system, multi-symptom illnesses acquired following exposure to environmentally produced biotoxins" (Shoemaker et al. 2). People with CIRS have a genetic pre-disposition in their immune system that makes them susceptible to this illness. This genetic inability to properly remove these damaging

---

6   A VCS test consists of a visual test which evaluates your ability to detect contrast at different frequencies and a questionnaire. See Appendix A for more information about what a VCS test is and where to find one.

biotoxins means they recirculate in a person's system, making them sicker and sicker (Beshara). CIRS can be caused by several different biotoxins (Lyme disease bacteria, ciguatera toxin, mold toxins, etc.), and one prevalent source of these biotoxins is indoor air in moist or water-damaged indoor environments. "Over 80% of CIRS cases reported stem from exposure to the interior environment of water-damaged buildings (WDB)" (Shoemaker et al. 13). Because it's a genetic susceptibility, there is no "cure" for CIRS at this time, but there is treatment through which the patient can regain their health and get rid of their symptoms.

The doctor's honesty and humility, and her taking the time to explain and direct me to resources where I could learn more, made me think, "Hmm... okay, I'll listen." She made no promises and didn't claim to know everything, but she made sure I could have access to as much information as possible. She was one of the most humble, honest, and respectful doctors I've seen. She even told me that she knows I've probably heard far too many doctors say that they could help me and that none of them did. She somehow knew what I'd been through and respected the gravity and impact of it, not expecting me to behave like I could, or should, trust her right off the bat.

After the second round of testing came back, I was diagnosed with CIRS. Though the knowledge of a new diagnosis didn't fill me with hope, there was something there... perhaps a spark... that I was afraid to even acknowledge because I didn't want to feel that horrible, crushing disappointment if this didn't work. But I'd finally found a doctor who I *might* be able to trust, and I was finally diagnosed with something that could explain *every single one* of the symptoms I'd been experiencing over the last several years.

Chapter 6

Treatment – The Attempt

*"Everything can be taken from a man except
one thing: the last of the human freedoms - to choose
one's attitude in any given set of circumstances,
to choose one's own way."*
- Viktor Frankl

The testing was extensive, detailed, and complex. But the doctor and her staff explained every result and what it meant. This was extremely helpful, especially when it came to the treatment for CIRS.

The first part of this treatment is removing the patient from exposure, and avoiding further exposure to these biotoxins and inflammatory triggers. Why? I've heard the reasoning explained by multiple doctors like this: Imagine you have a full bathtub and the plug is closed. The water represents the toxins. If the plug is removed – i.e. the medication to remove the toxins is taken – the water will drain and eventually be gone. However, if you turn the tap on – i.e. the patient remains in exposure, taking in these harmful toxins – even if you pull the plug, it will be anywhere from extremely difficult to impossible depending on the bathtub's ability to drain the water, i.e. the patient's ability to remove the toxins. That is why the very first step – the step deemed the most critical to a full recovery by all doctors who treat CIRS – is removing the patient from exposure and

the avoidance of re-exposure to these biotoxins and inflammatory triggers. Ultimately, this means remediating their current
environment (and its contents) to the standards for treatment,
or moving to a new environment that meets these standards
already, as well as avoiding re-exposure in the course of each
day, through their employment or school, appointments, and
any other activities outside their primary residence.

This part of treatment is difficult for some, but impossible
for others. The difficulty or impossibility is determined by a
number of factors. Obviously one factor is the ability to remediate or move, the availability of buildings/residences in their city
that meet the standards, as well as their employment/school
situation. The sensitivity of the patient is another factor because
it plays a large role in what it means to "sufficiently" remove
them from exposure. Though no environment is completely
free of toxins, there is a standard level of toxins considered ac-
ceptable for treatment when it comes to indoor environments.
And, though this works for the majority of CIRS patients, there
are those who are sensitive beyond this point or to inflammatory triggers that are not measured by any test available. So the
final say in whether a place is safe for the patient is really the
patient themselves (McMahon).

Another factor in a patient's sensitivity is how their body
reacts to each re-exposure. The reactions can vary widely.
Some patients can still recover despite living in and/or having
irregular exposures to environments that do not meet these
treatment standards. Then there are those who are more sensitive, who must live in an environment that meets or exceeds
treatment standards and just one exposure to an environment
that doesn't meet these standards can set back their progress
for weeks. Then, of course, there are those who lie in between
these two extremes to varying degrees.

With all this new knowledge in hand, and what was still
being learned, my parents and I began the search for a safe
place for me to live and progress through treatment. While we

searched for and tested potential living environments, I was fortunate to get to stay with a family friend who had a relatively new home with no carpet, that I didn't seem to react to. We tested several family members' homes, hoping I could stay with them. Testing consisted of collecting a dust sample and sending it into a specialized lab that analyzes the DNA of the sample by looking for 36 species of molds. It determines the levels of those species present, then assigns a score.[7] Surprisingly, each test came back falling far too short of the treatment standards and was on par with our own house. Next, we resorted to testing homes where people were renting out a room. First, we'd look for a listing of a newer home in the area. Then we'd reach out to the owner to see if they were open to a long-term stay, and we'd explain the circumstances. Then I'd visit to see how I felt. In a bad environment, within 15-20 minutes I tended to have symptoms like increased brain fog or neuropathy. So if I didn't have symptoms within those 15-20 minutes, we would take a dust sample and send it in for testing. I found that if I gave myself a few days to recover from each exposure that did cause symptoms to increase, then I would recover to my baseline and was able to tell if the next home made me worse or not. Despite my risking exposure to limit the number of tests and disappointments, the environments continued to fall far short of the requirements, just like the ones before.

---

7   The testing gives two scores: an ERMI score and a HERTSMI-2 score. They both use a genetic sequencing of the DNA of mold species to determine the spore equivalents per gram of dust and apply an index score. ERMI (Environmental Relative Moldiness Index) was based upon studies of childhood asthma and buildings done by the HUD in 2006. The HERTSMI-2 (Health Effects Roster of Type-Specific Formers of Mycotoxins and Inflammagens - 2nd version) is a weighted score designed by CIRS researchers to determine a level that is safe for patients with CIRS. "Generally, HERTSMI-2 is far superior to predict exposure safety. Due to the math calculation for the ERMI, the score may be skewed by a number of irrelevant organisms" (Dooley). Both indices are used as a guide; it is the patient's symptoms and lab results that ultimately determine the safety of a building.

In the meantime, I had been staying with our family friend for quite some time, and I had started treatment for giardiasis, which had made its way into my weakened and vulnerable gut. The treatment hit my body hard, but it was only a three-day regimen. So my mom would come and take care of me during those three days, and our family friend was kind enough to help care for me as well. But immediately after that three-day treatment, I began the treatment for another gut infection and took a turn for the worse. I began having episodes where I could barely walk or move my limbs, I was having trouble forming words and speaking, and I was in excruciating pain. So our family friend called my mom, who rushed over, and we went straight to the Urgent Care. The drive there was surreal. I would have expected to be afraid, but despite the spaciness of my thoughts and being too weak to support my own body, I wasn't freaking out or spiraling into anxiety; I was calm. When we arrived, both my mom and our friend had to support me so I could stand and walk to the front door of the Urgent Care center. At the door, I suddenly lost all control of my body and collapsed. My head flopped back and my body went limp. I was later told that, when the Urgent Care team witnessed this, they immediately said they couldn't treat me there and called an ambulance.

In the ambulance, on the way to the ER, I remember one of the EMTs tapping me and reminding me to breathe. I had to concentrate to take a breath when he said that. Once at the ER, I started to come out of the episode a little bit and was able to gently move my limbs, though I still felt weak. The doctor came in to tell us that my vitals had been stable, and they were going to run more tests. After the tests came back normal, the ER doctor basically said that they would release me and that was it. They didn't know what had happened. But, while we were waiting in the room to be released, I suddenly began to feel whatever had happened before, happening again. I felt really hot, then as if I was fading away; I couldn't move my arms and legs, then I couldn't speak, I couldn't think. Before I was completely in the episode, my mom recalled that I said, "Mom, I don't feel so well," and then my eyes rolled back. My mom went out to the nurse's station, telling the nurse there that whatever happened to me was happening again. A nurse came in and put me on oxygen while she went to get the doctor, but it took the doctor over ten minutes to get there and, by that time, I began to come out of whatever it was. Like before, she said that everything was stable and took me off the oxygen saying, "Who put this on her? She doesn't need this."

By this point I still couldn't speak, but I was aware of what was going on around me, and I remember the doctor asking my mom, "Does she have a history of anxiety?" I didn't have the ability to express how much this pissed me off, but my mom did. My mom is not one for confrontation, but she scoffed and laughed out loud, not being able to help her reaction to the doctor's cliché response to a condition like mine. My mom later told me that the doctor's eyes got really big, and her demeanor changed. My mom explained to her that her insinuation of anxiety happens so often to people who have conditions like mine, that it is considered a cliché that we joke about. Surprisingly, the doctor became receptive and actually took down the information my mom gave her on where she could find more information on CIRS. I was lucky in that this was the first doctor to suggest a psychological cause for my condition and health issues. Even so, I remember how invalidating this felt and how I wished I was able to speak at the time and say, "Yes, I have had anxiety attacks and panic attacks, and this is not that."

We later consulted with my functional medicine doctor, who conjectured that this reaction could have been a die-off reaction, where my body was overwhelmed trying to clean up the leftover bits from the organisms we were killing off.

Regardless, after I ended up in the ER, it became clear that I would need more regular and vigilant care to continue treatment, which meant my family needed around-the-clock access. So I moved into the first floor of a month-old motel so my parents could easily come and go as I needed them. We knew I couldn't stay there forever, but we seemed to be getting nowhere with homes that rented out a room. Becoming desperate as my health began to decline, we had to switch gears and start testing apartments. We used the same technique. We limited our search to the newest apartments available, and used me as a human mold detector. This was clearly not ideal, as I had to put myself at risk of getting sick, and often did get sick. But each test was $240-$300 and took a week or two to come back. We had already spent over $1,200 on testing with nothing to show for it (except a broader understanding of the state of buildings in Houston), all while we treated the intestinal issues (which also proved costly), and we were about to invest in my staying at a newly built apartment for who knows how long. So I did what had to be done so we could financially sustain treatment and all the costs of finding a safe place to live.

Though the motel was brand new, it was not well built, leaving it vulnerable to daily water damage, and I was getting sicker the longer I stayed. But even the brand new apartments we were looking at caused symptoms or had visible issues that would cause or had already caused water damage. So, when we found a 1-2 year-old apartment that didn't seem to increase my symptoms and tested better than anything we had seen so far – despite the fact that it did not quite meet treatment standards – we jumped on it, thinking it was better than the alternative.

Slightly adjusting the treatment protocol, my doctor had me start the second stage of treatment while we searched for a safe place for me to live. The second stage is taking an oral medication referred to as a "binder" that does what the majority of people's bodies do naturally and binds to the toxins, allowing them to be removed from the body. Once I moved into the somewhat-CIRS-safe apartment, and we had brought in only the non-porous items and things that could be cleaned, I began to further increase my use and dosage of this binder.

Then, being out of the toxin-heavy environments and on this second part of the treatment, I began to see progress to the point where I could more regularly care for myself, which became critical, living alone in that apartment 25 minutes away from my family.

In the beginning, living alone was very difficult because I had no car, I almost never had visitors, and caring for myself was a daily struggle. On good days, I could prepare my own food, wash up after, and do my laundry, punctuated by rest periods in between. Still, at the end of the day, I'd struggle to get myself to simply brush my teeth and take out my contact lenses before going to bed. During bad spells, I could hardly get out of bed or sit up to eat. My mom or dad could come once or twice a day for a few hours and prepare food and wash dishes, but the rest of the day I was on my own.

During this time I was also adding more supplements to help with methylation which, because my body was so inflamed, ended up causing anxiety, depression, and mood swings. On top of these chemically-induced emotions, I had the emotional stress of having a long-overdue confrontation of the suppressed attraction and feeling that existed between myself and a childhood friend. When that didn't end well, I lost a close friend who I thought would be in my life forever. At that time, I think he may have been that last bit of my old life, before I was sick, that I was desperately holding onto, fighting the fact that my life had been dramatically and irreversibly changed. I felt isolated, alone, and I was hurting – mind, body, and soul. I found myself yet again feeling broken and alone.

This is when I realized, if I am so broken and shattered, is this not the perfect time to rebuild myself into something more powerful, more beautiful than ever before? So that's exactly what I did. Every morning I listened to Tony Robbins and other motivational/self-help coaches and speakers on YouTube. I reached out to my mentors and drank in their advice and instruction. One such mentor, Don Akers, helped me learn how to listen to my body, which I never did when dancing as I almost always pushed through any pain or fatigue. Learning to listen to my body gave me the ability to take in all factors, like how I was feeling and what I needed to get done, in order to decide whether pushing through fatigue and pain would actually be beneficial. During this time, I learned to apply my stubbornness wisely, instead of impulsively without thought to the damage it might cause.

I listened, I learned, and I applied myself. Slowly, I began to see a strength grow from within me. I added tools to my metaphorical toolbox and used them to get through every day. I printed out my favorite quotes, laminated them, and put them up all over the apartment. I listened to my favorite music while going about my day so that my mind wouldn't be solely focused on the pain and fatigue. I learned to appreciate and feel gratitude for the little things like having running water, having food to eat, or seeing a sunset. Instead of focusing on feelings of loneliness, I found ways to relish living alone. I played whatever music I wanted when I wanted, walked around with as little clothes on as I pleased, and gave myself a schedule of cooking, resting, treatment, and anything else I was able to do, focusing on the fact that I was able to go about the day uninterrupted. Slowly I began to respect myself, my time, and what little energy I did have. So I stopped trying to hold on to people who clearly could not be the kind of friends I needed. I let go of people who hurt me and betrayed my trust. I let go of people who made me feel "less than". And I let in people who treated me with understanding, love, and respect. I let my family in, in ways I never had before. I enjoyed our time together like never before. I got out to meet the staff of the apartment and the neighbors whenever I could, and I made new friends that treated me with kindness and acceptance.

Though my emotional and mental fortitude flourished during this time, my physical health did not. It seemed the binder could not keep up with the influx of new toxins as well as get rid of the toxins stuck in my body from a lifetime of exposure. You see, living in humid, rainy, and moldy-as-hell Houston, nearly every building I went into made me sick, dialing up my neuropathy, pain, and cognitive symptoms.

Imagine that everywhere you go you are at risk of getting exposed to something that could make you feel sick for days, weeks, even months, and cause you significant pain. So you stay at home, where it's safe, except to get essentials. But even when you go out to get essentials, you're constantly on edge, afraid of what the environment you just entered could do to you. You can't go out with your friends to movies, or restaurants, or anything indoors, and you can't even do simple things like get your hair cut without taking a significant risk and likely becoming ill. This was what it was like living in Houston with CIRS. I was constantly aware of this, fearing exposure every time I went out because the consequences could be painful and debilitating. Eventually, I stopped trying to go anywhere but the grocery store for essentials, doctor visits only as absolutely necessary, and outdoors just to get out (despite the Houston heat and mosquitoes, who seemed to like my blood especially). Because I could not escape from exposure and because my living environment was, to an extent, additional exposure, the binder couldn't keep up. The tub couldn't drain.

On top of that, after about six months on the pharmaceutical binder, my body seemed to no longer tolerate it. The pain in my stomach was excruciating. It kept me up at night; or if I was asleep, I'd wake in the middle of the night crying out in pain and clutching my abdomen. It got so bad that I ended up in Urgent Care, nearly having to go to the ER for a second time during treatment. So I had to stop taking that binder. And, once I did, I began to see a decline in the progress I had made.

This severe stomach pain persisted even after I stopped the binder, which meant going into a doctor's office, which meant more exposure. I tried to handle this the best I could to avoid as much exposure as possible. I asked if they could see me outside, but they said they couldn't due to "insurance reasons". So I instead waited outside while my mom sat in the waiting room until they were ready to call me back. One appointment, even knowing my sensitivity to the building, they called me to come inside but I still ended up having to wait 45 minutes inside before I actually saw the doctor. And that office was bad. I could smell the mustiness and feel the brain fog, neuropathy, and dysautonomia increasing the longer I stayed, despite wearing an N95 mask. Because of the very stomach issues I was there for, I couldn't even take the prescription binder to combat this. It took me months to recover back to my previous baseline from the full hour of exposure from that one appointment.

Because I was this sensitive, and because Houston buildings were generally so moldy, completing the first step of treatment while there proved impossible. If the first step was to get out of exposure, both in my home and daily exposures, how could I possibly move on to Step 2 while in Houston? Even if my family could find a way to afford to build a brand new house, there was no guarantee of if or how long it would be safe for me. And there was no way for me to manage the impacts of the air quality in the environments which I had no control over, like stores, doctors' offices, and any other places I visited regularly. At this impasse, my doctor suggested I consider moving to a drier climate with less rain and humidity, like a desert. The dryness would perhaps make mold, and therefore its toxic byproducts, less prevalent in indoor environments.

The idea of moving again was daunting. I had been moving from place to place, living out of plastic bags for nearly a year. Every time I moved, I had to clean all my belongings per the protocol before they could be brought into the new environment. And it felt like, as soon as I got unpacked, settled, and comfortable somewhere, I had to move again and do the whole process all over again. On top of this, moving somewhere all alone where I knew no one was a scary thought for both me and my parents, not to mention impractical, since I wouldn't be able to take care of myself, drive, or work until I went through treatment. But by this time, my youngest brother's health had begun to decline significantly as well. He'd come in from playing outside or dancing saying, "My legs hurt," and would lie in bed for the rest of the day feeling sick. Despite previously dancing 10 hours a week, he began having trouble getting through a single dance class and was starting to have to sit out – getting dizzy and weak in the legs – until he was consistently only able to do about 45 minutes, twice a week. This progression was all too familiar, so my parents had him tested for the genetic susceptibility to CIRS. He had the exact same genetic variations that I have.

Additionally, because CIRS is genetic, when I learned of the cause of my illness, we realized that my mother, who had been dealing with chronic fatigue for more than six years, likely had it as well. So far, two out of the five of us had the genetic variation and the multi-system cluster of symptoms, and it was likely that my mother had it too. We realized that none of us could have a full, healthy life in Houston. So my family and I made the decision to get me out before I lapsed back into being completely unable to care for myself, and to get them out as soon as my brother finished his academic year.

It felt like a shot in the dark. It felt like a move of desperation. Was this really going to work? Were we sure we had pinpointed the root of our health problems? Though my mother was well-read on the condition and convinced of its validity, the Centers for Disease Control and Prevention (CDC) doesn't say anything about it, and your average internist or general practitioner can't diagnose it.[8] So it felt like a huge leap of faith for all of us.

---

8   See Appendix B: "Has CIRS Been 'Proven'?" for more information on this issue.

But now, through research and interviews with so many doctors that successfully treat CIRS, I've learned that there is a lot of research and literature that supports mold-induced illness. Though several things may contribute to CIRS not being widely accepted and acknowledged, one issue is that the idea of something "being proven" in the medical and scientific community seems to ultimately come down to a matter of opinion, which makes the most prevalent opinion the most accepted.

Of course, at the time of our decision to move, we knew none of this. But despite all the doubts and unknowns, with my family's financial and emotional support, we decided I would leave Houston for a drier climate as soon as possible, and they would follow. The research for a good place to move commenced. We discussed options in Utah, Nevada, Arizona, and Colorado – though we knew no one in any of these places. We ultimately decided that Arizona would be the best option for us to try to build a new life and find a safe home.

Chapter 7
The Move

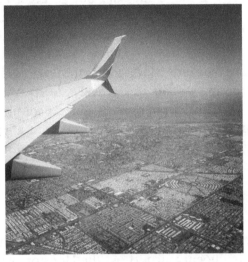

Photo from the plane descending into
Phoenix, AZ

Moving to Arizona was one of the best decisions in my life. But it certainly was not an easy task, even with the help and support of my family.

In the winter of 2018, my parents visited Arizona to be sure that it was a good choice for us, scout out the buildings, and to look at schools for my brothers. They rented a room in a house for a few nights, whereupon arriving they didn't smell mustiness, nor did my mom feel poorly there. They loved Arizona and noticed a huge difference in the indoor air quality of the buildings overall. But they knew: even being in the desert, there would still be buildings with mold growth. So when we considered where I would stay while looking for our future home, we figured it was best to go with something we were already familiar with. So, with the permission of the owner of the house my parents stayed in, we got it tested to make sure it would be safe for me, and bought my plane ticket to Arizona.

As happens in life, things did not go according to plan. There were mix-ups and mistakes in getting the house tested, and I boarded the plane not knowing if there would be a safe place for me to stay. However, I knew that I couldn't stay where I was. Without the binder, I was losing the progress I had gained and was becoming weaker and weaker. Clearly, treatment had begun to work, but I would not be able to continue it where I was. So, in March of 2019, I left Texas with a great deal of uncertainty. But I had something that I had not felt for quite some time: I had hope.

≡

I will never forget what it was like going from the Houston airport to the Phoenix airport. At the Houston airport, I was standing in line to board the plane, and I suddenly began to feel weaker, as though my legs might give out. I looked up and realized I was stuck under a vent. A/C units that are exposed to too much humidity tend to be breeding grounds for mold, so the fact that I was experiencing this under a vent in Houston was par for the course. I tried to move from under the vent by standing off to the side and slightly invading the personal space of the person in front of me.

When we finally boarded, I sat at a window seat, looking out at the overcast sky. When I felt the plane accelerate beneath me and we began to fly up and away from the dark fog of Houston, I felt my heart leap in my chest. Excitement and joy like I had not felt for years filled me up. There had been so much pain and suffering here, and I got to leave it all behind. The baggage of a long history of sickness and struggle. The person I used to be. The girl who constantly apologized and felt guilty for not conforming to the society that surrounded her in the suburbs of Houston. The girl who believed and acted as though she was weak and powerless. I left her behind when I left Texas.

The descent brought even more beautiful feelings of joy and freedom to the forefront of my mind. Clear skies revealed the rolling mountains and beautiful colors of the desert as we approached the landing strip. It was like flying into a paradise. In that moment, I knew this was a new beginning. Here, in Arizona, things would be different. I believed it and was determined to make it so.

When I stepped off the plane into the Phoenix airport, it was like stepping into a different world. The air smelled sweet. It was thin and pleasant to breathe, even inside the building.

One huge difficulty I had in Houston was having to find a bathroom to use all the time. Due to the dysregulation of the body's water balance caused by CIRS, sometimes I'd have to visit the bathroom multiple times within the span of an hour. So, even if I went out to a park or to do some other strictly outdoor activity, I would inevitably face the need to find a bathroom. Having poor ventilation and lots of moisture in a humid environment, bathrooms in Houston almost always made me feel sick. So, when I arrived in Arizona, I quite cautiously entered the ladies' room. But, to my surprise, the air didn't feel or smell any different in there. It wasn't stuffy and thick with the smell of mold like so many of the bathrooms in the Houston area. I couldn't believe it.

On the ride to the house where I'd be renting a room, I had a pleasant conversation with the driver and took in my surroundings. This is the desert? My eyes took in a stunning amount of green and a variety of plant species. I even saw palm trees! And the mountains –everywhere I looked I could see them standing powerful and beautiful like a landscape painting.

The roads were clean, without the dark dinginess of mud and mold I was accustomed to seeing. There were even sculptures and murals on the sides of the highways. I'll admit, perhaps my mind and the hope in my heart amplified the beauty of what I saw, but there was certainly plenty of beauty to be amplified.

Yet when I arrived at the house, I could feel that the air inside wasn't so great. It wasn't the worst either, so I withheld judgment – and panic. After introductions were made and the tour was given, I commenced the tedious task of cleaning every one of my belongings from my three suitcases. Washables went in the washing machine with borax, and I wiped down everything else with Decon-30.[9] Despite not yet having the test results, our belief was that this was a safer environment than where I came from, so I had to clean everything to make sure I wasn't bringing any of the toxins from the environment I was in previously to my new environment.

During the beginning of my stay at the rental, I noticed that I wasn't really getting any worse, but I also wasn't getting any better despite continuing treatment with an alternative binder. Eventually, we got the results of the test and discovered that, though it was better than most places we had tested in Houston, it too was not up to treatment standards. This confirmation of my suspicion put even more of a flame under my tiny tush to find a safe place for my family and me to live. In the meantime, I spent as much time as possible outside, or next to my air purifier.

The search for a safe home was, to be honest, quite depressing. Luckily, I was able to work with an agent who was patient and attentive in helping me find a house that could meet the necessary standards. But despite this, so many of the houses I looked at, I knew as soon as I entered them that they would not

---

9   Decon-30, a product by Benefect', is the cleaner that my family and I came across in our reading that was recommended for CIRS patients. There may be other products out there that are just as effective, but this is the one I use.

be safe. This came as a shock because I thought we'd have much better luck with houses in Arizona. Eventually we found one that didn't immediately make me sick, so I gathered a sample and rushed it to the lab. A week later the results came back, again, better than what we had seen in Houston, but not up to standards. So the search continued. At last, I found a house that didn't make me sick, and the test results finally came back with good news! But as we feared, before we were even able to get the results back, the house was rented to someone else. Despite paying for overnight delivery to the lab, and a rush on the test, the delay of having to wait for results proved to be a delay that cost us having a safe home.

At this point, I was running out of time before my family would arrive, and the environment of the house I was renting a room in was beginning to cause my health to regress. On top of this, I ended up getting very sick during my stay. I ran a high fever, my sinuses were clogged up, I was having severe nausea and vomiting, and all of my symptoms increased. During this time, I was unable to do even the basics of caring for myself, and we had to hire a home health nurse. In about a week I recovered, but not fully. I was still having trouble keeping up with taking care of myself and keeping the common spaces clean after cooking. I would cook, rest in the adjacent living room, and then clean. But the owner of the home insisted that the kitchen be cleaned immediately after cooking. With my body's inability to recover back to my baseline where I could meet these standards, it became clear that I needed to find a safe place to live where I could rest as needed and go at the pace my body required.

We were also starting to fear what would happen if we were locked into a 12-month lease in a house that experienced water damage. Would the owner take care of it properly? So we decided to abandon our search for a house and start looking at apartments. An apartment with a short lease term seemed like the least risky solution. My parents did the research, and I did the visiting. We tried to keep our search to newer developments so we weren't paying for as many tests, and so I wasn't risking too much exposure.

After visiting a handful of developments, we finally found one – and what a find this was! Technically speaking, even this apartment was not perfectly up to the standards as we understood them at the time. But it was so close – the closest we had ever seen – so we decided to take it. I packed all of my things in my three suitcases and booked a ride-share to the apartment. We got a mattress shipped there, and I bunked on the mattress on the floor until my family made it there with all the other belongings and non-porous furniture. I started the cleaning process while on my own – once again wiping down *every* item with Decon-30 – and once my family arrived, we worked together. Every single household item that we could keep was either wiped down on the patio, laundered multiple times, or put through the dishwasher. Painstakingly, over months, we worked our way through every single box. But we were finally somewhere safe. And, finally, nearly a year after being diagnosed, I was able to truly undertake treatment.

Chapter 8
Treatment – For Real This Time

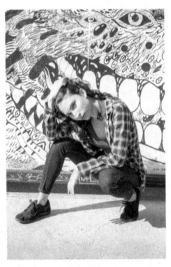

Viviane Lovato
Photo by JJ Hart (2019)

As soon as I moved into the apartment in May of 2019, I started treatment again. My stomach still couldn't tolerate the original binder, so we had to experiment with other binders to get the toxins out of my body. These binders were not as potent or proven, but the alternative was too painful, and potentially dangerous. So we gave every other option a shot.

After a few weeks, I began to see real progress. At last! By the end of summer in 2019, I was doing yoga every other day and workouts on the days I didn't do yoga. Sometimes,

I'd even walk down to the basketball court and freestyle dance for however much time I could handle. It was such a joy to be able to work out and dance again. Not only that, I was making new friends and going out almost every weekend. I was lucky enough to find a group of friends who accepted that I couldn't necessarily just go anywhere, and they were always supportive when I told them I couldn't stay in a building that was making me sick.

Though there were still buildings that made me sick, I found that it was only around half of the buildings. This allowed me so much more freedom than I had in Houston, where I'd say about 98% of the buildings I went into made me sick. I was finally able to get a haircut, go to the movies, go to a museum; I even got to go clubbing – one of my favorite social activities. I was still living with the pain and fatigue, but the fact that I could exercise again and had a social life was huge.

But just as things were finally improving, there was water damage in the apartment above us... which meant water damage in our ceiling. My mom was the first to catch it. She spotted the watermarks on our ceiling and immediately reached out to maintenance. As soon as possible, the apartment complex got a remediator to come in. The trouble is, most remediators don't know about CIRS or how to remediate at the necessary level for CIRS patients. My mom had to educate the remediator on CIRS and biotoxins so that he could take the necessary precautions to keep the toxins from spreading, and so that he could remediate our apartment per our specific health needs.

At first, the remediator was dismissive, confident in his knowledge and his training, unaware that there was more to be learned. He just did not seem receptive to the information my mom was giving him. But he seemed to have a good rapport with my dad. My dad, realizing this, had a conversation in passing with the remediator. He told him how my mom is the one who's done all the research on CIRS for the family, so she's the one to get information from. He also mentioned her history as an engineer in order to demonstrate that she is, in fact, an educated woman with two college degrees and real-world experience. To further convince the remediator of the value of this information, my dad appealed to his business nature and explained that this was a huge business opportunity for any remediator. My dad told him that a shift in understanding was coming and, being business-minded himself, if he were the remediator, he would learn everything he could on how to meet this particular health condition's needs.

After this conversation, the remediator became much more receptive and curious. My mom sent him an article from an online source for indoor environmental professionals (IEPs) and remediators, and she worked closely with him through the remediation process – explaining, teaching, and informing throughout. He listened, learned, and applied, accommodating our special needs as best he could with the tools he had, even using some of the tools we had, like our air purifier meant specifically to capture those extremely small particulates that are harmful to those of us with CIRS.

Because of the location of the water damage, the A/C system had to be shut off. It was summer in Arizona, so there was no way we could all stay in the apartment while it underwent remediation. The apartment complex paid for a hotel for us all to stay in while the work was being done. We went to the hotel, hoping that I would feel okay there so we wouldn't have to figure out somewhere else for me to stay. But we weren't that lucky. After about 15 minutes in the hotel, I began feeling ill. There was another, more expensive but newer hotel nearby, so I stayed there for that night until we could figure something else out.

Traumatized by experiences with moldy environments in the past and fearful of losing all the progress I had made, I decided that the A/C-less apartment was the lesser of two evils. It was rough, but it wasn't all that bad. I drank lots of water, had lots of fans going, and managed the heat in any other way I could think of.

When it was finally finished, we cleaned the contained area per the treatment protocol, moved back in, and waited to gather dust to test the apartment again. The test results came back not quite as good as before, but they were still good enough. So, for now at least, we still had a safe place to live. But this unexpected event and all we had to go through because of it, brought into sharp relief the reality that we're always one water-damage event away from being displaced.

I continued treatment through this whole debacle, but some components had to be halted, so I picked those up right where I left off when it was over. To get a more objective measure of the level of toxins in my body, I took a Visual Contrast Sensitivity (VCS) test before every appointment with my doctor, who continued to treat me via telemedicine after I moved from Texas. The VCS tests showed that, despite the progress we were seeing, my toxin levels were still too high. When I was still failing the VCS test – after nearly two years of trying to pass – in the fall of 2019, my doctor agreed I should try doing the next stage of treatment and see if that helped to get the level of toxins down.

The next stage of treatment, in my case, was the eradication of MARCoNS (Multiple Antibiotic Resistant Coagulase Negative Staphylococci), bacteria that take up residence in the nasal passageways of many CIRS patients and can cause a number of symptoms – physical, cognitive, and psychological. The seemingly simple treatment involves regular use of a specially-made nasal spray for a prescribed period of time. I had tried to start this treatment a couple of times in Houston, but my body was unable to tolerate it. I was hit so hard with pain, crushing fatigue, dizziness, weakness, and psychological symptoms that I was struggling to care for myself and was getting dangerously close to winding up in the ER again. With what I had experienced with this treatment before, I was very scared to try it again, but it seemed I was out of options. So I gathered my courage, all the tools I'd collected throughout the years to get through times like this, the support of my family, and I commenced the 102-day treatment for MARCoNS.

≡

The first month of MARCoNS treatment was a challenge, to say the least. Nearly immediately after starting it, I was dealing with full-on fatigue, fibromyalgia, dysautonomia, neuropathy, etc. – all over again.

I was unable to continue my workouts and spent most of the early days of treatment lying down. It really messed with my head. Not only was it hard to be feeling so sick again, but there were psychological symptoms as well. The OCD, which had become less and less debilitating the more I went through CIRS treatment, went back to being as disruptive as it was before I left Houston, and I had episodes of depression, anxiety, and irritability. Luckily, I had experienced these kinds of psychological symptoms before and was able to relatively quickly identify the fact that they were indeed symptoms, what I label "chemical emotions", and not emotions coming from any real dissatisfaction or despair in my life. This knowledge helped to take power away from the thoughts that these symptoms brought on, especially when it came to depression.

My family was also a huge help; they were incredibly patient and supportive through this time. But their patience was tried at times. Sometimes, out of nowhere, I'd get extremely irritable and the smallest things would set me off. Other times, I'd suddenly shut down and get really depressed. The OCD would cause me to freak out, for example, when they put something of mine down somewhere the germaphobia-OCD had deemed dirty. My OCD had gotten so much better that these kinds of reactions were a bit of a shock to us all, but during this time, my family went back to not moving any of my things without my permission. They acted with understanding to the best of their ability and accepted that I was doing my very best to handle and manage these symptoms. And we got through it.

I found as many ways as I could to be productive during this time to combat the "chemical emotions" and feelings of stagnation. I watched movies in Spanish (a language I'd been trying to learn for years), I dedicated myself to eating right and taking my medication, and I reminded myself that every day was a step closer to healing and health. I'd mark off the days on my calendar, feeling a sense of pride for getting through each day as I marked it off. Midway through the treatment, I was able to do some stretching and maybe a walk on the good days, which truly helped my moods. So I added what I could and continued counting down the days. Eventually, toward the very end of the treatment, I was able to freestyle on some days and stretch on others. This made getting through each day a lot easier, as dance has always been my best and favorite tool for processing, letting go of emotions, having fun, and just generally feeling good.

Finally, in February of 2020, I finished the allotted time for MARCoNS treatment. I took a nasal swab test to see if I had fully eradicated those nasty bacteria. The results came back negative, and I was finally able to move on to the next part of treatment!

Up until this point, I had been doing treatment to get rid of or kill off invaders my body had been exposed to when made vulnerable by CIRS. And, because my body seems to have such a hard time "cleaning house", this part of the treatment was extremely tough for me. But it was finally time to rebuild, repair, and give my body what it could not give itself. It was finally time to do treatment that would make me feel better – maybe better than I can ever remember feeling.

Chapter 9
Healing and Headway

"It's not whether you get knocked down.
It is whether you get back up again."
- Vince Lombardi

When I first started the gentler process of repairing and complementing my body, I did feel better than I had in years. I was able to exercise every day and work on the writing and transcription business I was building to support myself financially. I started dancing so regularly throughout the week that neighbors began to come by and watch on the days I'd go out. For the first time in years, I was not having to constantly ration my energy; I was flying through the days.

That lasted for about three weeks. After being unknowingly re-exposed to biotoxins, I found myself in a crash, feeling poorly, again.

But what was the source? This question is often answered through trial and error. One source of this exposure turned out to be a blanket we had brought from Houston. We had cleaned it per the protocol several times, and I had started using it outside to shield myself from the sun while I did yoga on the balcony. But, for whatever reason, this material seemed to retain the particles from our old environment. The solution was simple: we threw the blanket out.

Another possible source we discovered was the car we had from Houston, which I had started driving more often as I had begun to feel better. Once I realized this could be a source of exposure, I decided to see how I felt when I drove it and when I didn't, which led to the discovery that it was indeed affecting me. My parents had cleaned and vacuumed the car upon their arrival in Arizona, but apparently this wasn't enough. So they went even deeper in their cleaning method. They cleared everything out, cleaned and shampooed the carpet with another Benefect® product, and ran one of the air purifiers from our apartment in the car while they had the A/C running. Afterward, even they noticed an improvement in the air quality in the car, and thankfully I found that I no longer seemed to react to it.

The crash that resulted from these two exposures was less debilitating than most I've had before, and I seemed to recover faster than I ever had before. This was progress! If I was seeing a less severe reaction to inflammagens already, maybe there was hope for even less reactivity in my future. After about three weeks spent recovering, I neared the level of activity I was doing before. And a few weeks later, I was back to feeling better than I have in years. Not only that, I seemed to be feeling *that* good more and more consistently. For the first time in years, I found myself thinking about prioritizing things because I was running out of *time,* instead of prioritizing things because I was running out of *energy.*

I could do a full hour of yoga, come straight inside to take a shower, and then clean up in the kitchen. Though my legs were a bit tired and I felt some pain, I didn't feel like I needed to go immediately lie down. This kind of activity, one after the other without consequences, was something I hadn't been able to do for years. Previously, when I did anything too physically or emotionally taxing, I'd find myself in a crash from pushing too hard. This is referred to as "push-crash syndrome" in patients who deal with exertion intolerance from chronic fatigue. So being able to go from one thing right to another after so many years of rationing my energy and fearing the push-crash cycle was so incredibly empowering.

When I found myself consistently doing yoga, dancing, and visualizing ballet classes in my mind, I realized it was finally time. Finally time to build my body and strengthen my muscles to go back to ballet. I had a plan and a structure for coming back. I wanted to start working out at the apartment's gym to build stamina and intended to see a physical therapist to help fix some of the issues I struggled with before I stopped dancing. But, as it was the spring of 2020, COVID-19 happened. So, like everyone else, I had to find ways to accomplish my goals without the tools I thought I'd have.

This wasn't the first time I've had to make do with the inability to go anywhere, so that aspect didn't faze me much.

I looked back at notes I had taken over my previous years of dancing and searched for conditioning and strengthening exercises. I found the ones that targeted specific muscles I needed to bring my body back to being ballet ready, and the ones that address the issues I had hoped to fix with a physical therapist's guidance. I did these exercises daily, yoga three days a week to gain flexibility, and some form of dancing at least three times a week to gain stamina. Every day, I practiced some foundational ballet moves with special attention to those muscles I'd been retraining and rebuilding. By the summer of 2020, I began learning choreography and combinations using not only my mind but my body as well. I even participated in a world-wide virtual choreography project!

Also at this time, my mom and brother had been improving and getting treated. When they arrived in Arizona, my brother saw massive improvement, even without the care of a doctor, as some CIRS patients do. He went from being unable to tolerate dancing less than an hour at the studio in Houston, to doing summer training here in Arizona that involved six hours of dancing a day, five days a week. Then, in the fall of 2019, he continued to do rigorous dance training as well as his academics, with none of the fatigue issues he had in Houston. My mom saw some improvement in her health, but it wasn't until she started getting treated by a functional medicine and CIRS-certified doctor that she began to see true improvement. She went from being so ill, struggling to get through every day, to being able to go out walking, swimming, or on short hikes. She had bad days, and she still experienced push-crash syndrome. But she wasn't far into treatment yet. So I was excited that, even at the beginning of treatment, she was starting to have better days, sometimes even good ones.

I also began discovering and dedicating myself to advocacy for CIRS. It was suggested to me around this time that I take the time to write about my experiences. I decided that if I was going to do this, I would write about my journey and direct people to a place that helps people with CIRS. The more I searched, the more I realized just how much and what is needed to help people who are struggling with CIRS. And the more I learned about it, the more I began to see that I might have a place in this. I began to see that, even now as a 21-year-old whose sole accomplishment has been surviving CIRS, I may have the ability, potential, and resources to make a difference.

≡

Everything was taking off for me and my family. And, for the first time in years, I felt like I was getting to progress in my life, not just in my health. But the challenges kept coming.

In June of 2020, somehow I sprained ligaments in my lower back when I walked into the corner of the kitchen counter, slamming my hip bone and falling to the floor. It took over two months to recover from the injury and, during those two months, I had to dig deep for patience and strength.

I learned that low vascular endothelial growth factor (VEGF) greatly contributed to my body's structure being so fragile and taking so long to heal.[10] So I began to target this issue with the help of physical therapy and the last step of the CIRS protocol, a medicine called VIP (vasoactive intestinal peptide). I determined to keep my body's fragility in mind and to continue to do exercises to strengthen the parts of my body that are weak.

I also started listening to Tony Robbins again every morning. I found interviews he did with successful people who came from humble beginnings, and I drew inspiration and strength from their stories. I also asked myself the question, "How can I make this setback work for me?" This is when I realized something about my life and what it has taught me.

I realized that I have faced so many consecutive setbacks that have persisted for so long, that I've had to adjust the way I look at and handle them. If I allowed every setback to be a setback, I wouldn't make it very far. So, with every one, I've had to find ways to make them work for me. Each one is different, so my approach to each has been different. But the general principle remains the same: "What can I learn from this, and how can I make it work for me?"

How could I make this setback work for me? Well, I had all this time that I would have been using to dance or do yoga. So I needed to find other productive ways to use the time this injury had opened up for me. Writing my story, taking care of my injury, and doing exercises to strengthen my feet became my main focus for eight weeks after the injury. Because sitting was painful, I found ways to work on the computer standing up and lying down. I iced, did my physical therapy exercises, and stayed vigilant with my treatments. Studying dance videos and strengthening my feet were the only dance-related things I could do while injured, so I just focused on those and reminded

---

10   VEGF "stimulates new blood vessel formation and increases blood flow"; without this, cells "begin to starve and don't work properly"(Surviving Mold).

myself how each thing would eventually make me a better dancer.

But sometimes these setbacks come in waves, and healing from CIRS is a complicated and non-linear process full of unknowns and trial and error. While dealing with this injury, I had begun to get fatigue, fibromyalgia, dizziness, and muscle weakness. Again. And my mom was also having an increase in her symptoms. Seeing some concerning signs around the shower walls, and worried that hidden water damage was causing our increasing symptoms, our first step was to have a remediator come investigate with a moisture meter. He didn't find any red flags, so we decided to do some environmental testing used in CIRS treatment, ERMI and HERTSMI-2, to be sure that there wasn't anything hidden.

While this may seem like overkill, we did what's recommended for CIRS patients. Water damage and mold, especially at the low level that CIRS patients are sensitive to, can hide in the A/C units, the walls, and the floors, and can go undetected by the methods of investigation used by most mold inspectors, indoor environmental professionals (IEPs), and remediators.

While we waited for the investigation to complete and for the environmental test results, I had to pause my treatment. It is critical that VIP be taken in a safe environment. If one is exposed to biotoxins regularly during this treatment, it pretty much does the opposite of what it's supposed to do. So I had to be 100% sure that there wasn't any water damage in the apartment before continuing. And to our surprise and relief, the test results came back better than ever before.

Now that we had eliminated our home as a possible cause for our increase in symptoms, my mom and I turned our attention to our treatment, reasoning that something new there may actually be the source of our recent worsening of symptoms. On my end, I learned that a reaction to the turmeric that I had added for pain and inflammation from the back injury was likely causing my increased symptoms, and when I stopped that, my fibromyalgia pain began to fade, and I began to feel less fatigued. On my mom's end, she removed a couple of new things from her protocol, and she was able to isolate the problem as well.

It was throughout this time that one hard truth became clear to me: this won't be easy. I knew that. But I think, somewhere in the back of my mind, I thought that once I finally started getting better, everything would just fall into place. I guess I thought that I had earned that. And maybe things *will* fall into place at some point; maybe it will get easier and my health will be less fragile. Maybe one day I won't be constantly on alert, anticipating new water damage. I will certainly never stop striving for my optimum health so that I can get where I want to go and live my best life. But now I recognize that it will be one hell of a journey, and I've got no idea what the road will look like.

Ideally, even after completing treatment, I should be living in a CIRS-safe environment so that I have less reactivity to exposure outside of the home where I don't have control over the air quality. However, at this point in time, CIRS-safe housing – that will *stay* safe – isn't very accessible. Unless you count camping, as many CIRS patients do live out of a tent or their car, but let's be real, what kind of life and stability do these people have long-term? If you're *really* into camping, maybe it'd be nice. But it's definitely not the quality of life that most people desire. Technically, those living out of tents or their cars due to CIRS are homeless; made homeless by medical needs, so perhaps medically-induced homelessness, but they are still without a secure and reliable living situation.

As far as my career, I know I want to dance; I know I want to advocate for CIRS patients. But, with all the dangers that remain for sensitive CIRS patients, I'm forced to acknowledge that I'm not 100% sure what that will look like for me.

Chapter 10
The Future

*"Intense desire allows people to win
against overwhelming odds."*
- Ruben Gonzalez

After learning about CIRS and about my journey thus far, you may be thinking, "It's impossible. She can't have a career in dance. There's no way someone can do something like that with her condition."

And you may be partially right. The vision I had before for my life – joining a large company and rising up the ranks to principal dancer, maybe with a typical side job so that I can live comfortably on a dancer's salary – may no longer be feasible.

This would scare the hell out of me and make me want to curl up in a ball and hide from the world, ashamed that I can't live this picture-perfect life I had planned, convinced I'm doomed to be unhappy. But recent experiences have shown me that I shouldn't assume to know myself or what I want so completely and accurately.

Once, I had a relationship that was what I *thought* I wanted. And then, I had a friendship, romance, and love that filled my heart in ways I didn't know a relationship could. It broke all my rules and gave me everything I thought I didn't want and everything I thought I couldn't have. It opened my mind to see

I'm capable of more than I thought and that I could want these things I had determined were not for me.

Sadly, it could not continue, but even so, I feel lucky to have had this experience. So much about it remains a mystery to me, and I don't know exactly in how many and in what ways it has impacted me, my life, and my perception of these. But I do know it showed me that I need to be more open. I need to stop confining myself to some predetermined ideal. I need to follow where my passion and desires take me. When I do something and feel a pure happiness and feel like this is where I'm meant to be, I need to listen to that and accept it, not judge it and see if it fits some predetermined blueprint. I don't *really* know if that blueprint would in fact make me happy, and why should my life not fitting this blueprint matter, if what I am living right then and there *is* making me happy?

This experience was like the final shove into a newfound openness that has helped me to accept things that have come to a head over all these years. It's helped me to accept that the struggle – this painful growth – is far from over, that it may never be over, and that I don't know what my life will look like. But that's okay, because I can make something of this. I can still have a life of happiness and fulfillment, even if I don't know exactly how yet. I know I want to dance, and I know I want to use my experiences to help people suffering from CIRS. Who knows what vehicle or exact mechanism will be best for me and provide me the most happiness and fulfillment. As scary as the unknown is, it's also exciting and freeing to be open to new possibilities because I've stopped limiting myself to some predetermined plan and stopped kidding myself into thinking that I could somehow know what the future-me would want.

I will be honest with you, despite all the support I have, the progress I've made, and everything I've been through to get this far, sometimes I also doubt that I can do this. Sometimes I'm afraid of failing. Sometimes I'm afraid I'll settle for less than my dreams because pursuing them will be too challenging and too scary for a "control freak" trying to follow where her passion leads.

Then, I focus on and feel this fire inside me that just won't die; it's ignited by a purpose and a desire so strong that it's like a need. It creates a drive to succeed that's purer and stronger than ever. When I dance and when I fight for change for those like me, I'm truly happy and filled with purpose. When I am without these things, I feel their absence. I feel empty and purposeless, which leads my mind to dwell on the pain of things I've lost and the pain of past and present experiences that seem meaningless if I don't use them to create art and help others. Having dance and advocacy makes my life flow and feel naturally joyous. Having these things in my life just feels right.

The consequences of giving up, the gratitude I feel, the drive, and the joy I find in these things won't let me stop fighting; it won't let me settle or give up. Having this knowledge and focusing on these things gives me the power to push forward even as life continues to place challenges before me, and I believe it will continue to do so for as long as I allow it.

≡

As grateful as I am for the progress I've made and how lucky I am, I also recognize the reality of my condition and my situation. Though the fight to regain my health may be coming to a point where it isn't all-consuming, the fight to *maintain* my health while I pursue my goals and dreams is just beginning. In Arizona, I have a much better chance of succeeding in life and in my career than I did in Houston. However, even in Arizona, I've found I'm still negatively impacted by exposure to approximately 50% of the buildings. So any building I'm going to frequent will need to be tested; those that impact my health must be avoided. While my body may get stronger, and VIP might help lower my reactivity, and new advancements may be made, there's no guarantee these things will come to pass.

And, even if they do, I will likely still have to live and work in safe environments to maintain the health necessary to have an athletic career as a person whose body has been impacted by CIRS.

When the time comes, I'll need to find a safe place to live that I can afford on my own, which is incredibly difficult for a CIRS patient. And, as I've said before, CIRS-safe homes that *stay* CIRS-safe are just not accessible to most at this time, and newer developments that are more likely to be safe and stay safe for a period of time are usually quite expensive. This is one of the things that I hope to help progress and change, but accessible CIRS-safe housing probably won't be available when I regain my health and move out of my family's home. So where will I go?

And in order to dance professionally, or to get any job, I will need to test the buildings that I'll be working in regularly. As you may recall, testing is not cheap; it's upwards of $240 per test and must be done regularly to safeguard my health.

Even if I find ways around these things, it helps me get closer to where I want to go, but it doesn't solve the real problem. It doesn't confront the root of the problems that I will continue to face as I go through life, and that so many others with CIRS are facing today.

Chapter 11

Hurdles

So what is the root of the problems that CIRS patients face? Well, the truth is, it's more complex than just one root cause. But one large contributor to these problems is that there is very little in place to support and protect those with CIRS. So it is difficult to get a diagnosis and get through treatment, especially when it comes to finding or creating a safe home environment, keeping that home safe, and finding a safe work/school environment. And some never do.

First of all, there isn't an organization whose sole purpose is to advocate for the patient: to guide the patient through finding a doctor, finding a safe place to live and work, getting through treatment, and living a full life after treatment. And without a comprehensive advocacy organization, there also seems to be little protection and resources for patients.

That is not to say there are no resources at all. In addition to the multitude of blogs, personal journey stories, and ever-growing number of support groups that are online, there are two large organizations that educate about CIRS and environmentally acquired illness (EAI). Surviving Mold (survivingmold.com), for the most part, serves as a repository of information and studies on CIRS and directs patients to certified and proficient practitioners who are trained to recognize and diagnose it. The International Society for Environmentally Acquired Illness (iseai.org), while mostly geared toward practitioners, does have a robust list of support groups, articles, and a link to practitioners on their Patient Resources page. All of these sources – blogs, repositories, support groups, and personal stories – are very helpful. But one must have the mental and physical ability and stamina to find and sift through all these different sources, some more anecdotally-based and others more scientifically-based, and learn how to manage their condition themselves. This expectation to be your own advocate and expert is so well understood in the CIRS community, that in the 2018 diagnostic consensus statement, the authors said this of CIRS patients: "Outside learning will be included; one will probably be instructed to read several hundred pages of documents found (free) on www.survivingmold.com, understanding that few will remember everything. Most CIRS patients have difficulty assimilating new knowledge, but possibly loved ones will read and learn more as well. In time, patients must become an expert in the jargon and pathophysiology of CIRS" (Shoemaker et al. 4).

Understanding CIRS is complex in and of itself, and 90% or more of people with CIRS are dealing with not only physical illness but "some degree of brain fog (aka toxic encephalopathy)" (McMahon). For example, in my case, there was a long period of time when I was so ill that I could not tell my right from my left without concerted effort. Learning new things would require reading one sentence multiple times before fully comprehending it, and the effort would literally hurt my brain. And because of the complex and sometimes fatalistic way in which the information I was directed to was written, there was also the emotional toll of learning about it and thinking, "Holy sh--, this is my life now... my life is over."

Luckily, I had my doctor who directed me to important information and my mom who read, learned, and processed all the necessary information to form a plan and make the adjustments that inevitably arise through treatment. Often practitioners and family members are the only available resources of support, and some patients do not have the support of any family members. This leaves them with only their practitioners, who are already overwhelmed by treating, in some cases, thousands of patients. Dr. Ming Dooley who treats CIRS says, "I end up doing MUCH MUCH more for all my patients than I think most providers do as I know they won't get better without this."

Thankfully some headway is being made in the area of patient education. Dr. Sandeep Gupta and Caleb Rudd developed the *Mold Illness Made Simple* (MIMS) course that contributes to this. As a doctor who treats CIRS, Dr. Gupta got the "impression that a lot of the information on CIRS was far too complex for the person with CIRS to actually understand" (Gupta). He created this online course to help patients get a level of "calm and clarity" so that they can move forward with treatment and not be paralyzed by the diagnosis and treatment plan (Gupta).

I wish I had access to a course like this when I was first diagnosed with CIRS. In MIMS, Dr. Gupta goes over the basics of CIRS and CIRS treatment. He introduces the user to possible barriers throughout treatment and gives advice on possible ways to overcome these. Dr. Gupta does an incredible job of presenting the reality of living with CIRS without making the user feel like their life, or the life of their loved one, is virtually over. He is also very clear about when in the process of discovering CIRS a certified practitioner is needed. And he covers ways to navigate the current deficit of sufficiently educated IEPs and remediators when looking for a safe place to live/work or remediating a building. The course is geared towards patients and keeps in mind that common symptoms of CIRS include brain fog, fatigue, and poor tolerance of stress. So you can take it at your own pace.[11]

---

11 To access MIMS go to: www.moldillnessmadesimple.com?aff=vivianelovato (Disclosure: I will receive a portion of purchases made through this link).

Some people have a family member or loved one, like I did, who can help them. Or they can access a course to help them learn, digest, and implement the information given to them by their doctor. But many people are on their own. Because there isn't a place where resources are compiled and whose purpose is to guide these patients, each patient is getting access to different resources depending on what their doctor knows about. If their doctor doesn't know of some of these resources, like the MIMS course, they can't even suggest it to a patient. So, despite the resources being created, so many people are left having to search for information themselves (which leaves them vulnerable to bad information) or go only off of what their doctor is able to provide.

This information issue is a hurdle in and of itself but, even before this, the first hurdle to overcome is actually *finding* a doctor who can diagnose and treat you. I spent three years going from doctor to doctor, getting individual diagnoses without anyone understanding how they all fit together or what caused them in the first place. That makes me one of the lucky ones. "Based on the experience of thousands of initial office visits with CIRS providers it is likely that patients will have failed to find improvement from [at] least 10 physicians before, at least one of whom was a psychiatrist" (Shoemaker et al. 3).

Why do patients have to go to so many doctors for so long before getting a diagnosis? Lack of awareness and insufficient education greatly contribute to this phenomenon. Though these are both progressing, awareness and acknowledgment of CIRS are not commonplace. CIRS patients present with what the medical community calls "Medically Unexplained Symptoms (MUS)" (e.g. fibromyalgia, irritable bowel syndrome, chronic fatigue syndrome, etc.) resulting in many doctors seeing CIRS patients but being unaware that it is CIRS, which results in misdiagnosis (McMahon). And, even if you find a doctor who's aware of CIRS, "knowing about CIRS, doesn't necessarily mean capable of treating CIRS" (Dooley).

This is something that doctors and advocates across the globe are working to change, often without any outside funding, by highlighting and increasing the body of existing evidence and raising awareness. The literature review "A Comprehensive Review of Mold Literature Research from 2011-2018" highlights existing evidence. It is a result of a combined 1,500-plus unpaid hours of work by Dr. Ming Dooley and Dr. Scott McMahon. And it concludes that the "current literature supports multisystem adverse human health effects in those chronically exposed to indoor microbial growth/dampness" (Dooley and McMahon 2). This is just one example of the work being done by professionals working on CIRS with "ZERO dollars outside funding" (McMahon).[12]

Resources for guidance, information, and raising awareness – like the *Mold Illness Made Simple* course and many others – are constantly being generated by those in the field eager to help those suffering from CIRS. The certification process and *Proficiency Partners* course that doctors and practitioners can take to become knowledgeable of and qualified to help people with CIRS, created by Dr. Ritchie Shoemaker and his team, were huge leaps forward for awareness and acknowledgment of CIRS, and medical professionals are continuing to get trained through these courses.[13] But until your average general practitioner can recognize the signs of CIRS in their patients and refer them to practitioners who can further investigate and treat it, there is still so much to do.

The second hurdle, once you do find a doctor who is qualified to diagnose and treat CIRS[14], is how in the world to afford them. Most practitioners who specialize in CIRS do not

---

12   See Appendix B: "Has CIRS Been 'Proven'?" for more on this subject.

13   See Appendix A for more information on becoming qualified to treat CIRS.

14   See Appendix A for information on where to find these doctors.

accept insurance. To give the care necessary, CIRS doctors often spend hours on the first patient visit. For visits as long as this, in the insurance system, "time-based billing is the only option for which there are billing codes… The reimbursement [for the doctor] with such codes is abysmal" (McMahon). This system puts these practitioners in an impossible position. Dr. McMahon, a CIRS doctor at the forefront of promoting change for CIRS, put it this way: "Doctors that depend on insurance payments for a CIRS practice will go broke." If they do not rely on insurance payments, the burden then falls on the patient. As a self-pay patient, an initial visit can be well over $500, and each follow-up visit can be upwards of $300. And recovering from CIRS is not simple or straightforward; there is no single pill, diet, surgical procedure, or any one-off treatment. While there are exceptions, for most it takes time, and potentially years of office visits and medications. In addition to the appointments themselves, most of the medications used to treat CIRS currently have to be compounded. And, unless you have the rare insurance that is straightforward and simple in their coverage of compounded medication, this means additional effort to try to get it covered or high costs if you can't.

I was one of the lucky ones. I had a family who was willing to take the risk and use a significant portion of their savings – and had savings to use. Tragically, I know several friends and family members who have complex multi-system symptoms like mine and live in areas with lots of water-damaged buildings, but they just don't have the financial support to get any help.

So hurdle number three: if you do find a doctor, are diagnosed with CIRS, and can afford the visits and treatment, then you must accomplish the very first step of treatment – removal from exposure. There's really no way around this one. I've interviewed several CIRS certified doctors and practitioners, and all have reiterated what my doctor told me: the patient cannot fully regain their health and, as doctors, they cannot truly do their job, unless the patient is removed from exposure to the inflammagens that are making them sick. While doctors have seen some success in targeting other issues while doing the best they can with a poor environment, full recovery remains out of reach unless the patient is able to get out of the exposure.

My experience was a great example of this. My doctor was able to treat some of the effects of CIRS, like parasites and infections that can gain entry into a weakened body, while I was in a slightly improved environment in Houston. But much of this treatment resulted in a visit to the ER or Urgent Care because my body could not handle this stress while overrun by inflammatory toxins. And I couldn't rid my body of these toxins while in Houston, because the medication meant to do so could not keep up with the influx of new toxins I was exposed to every day.

Further complicating this step, it is statistically likely that you will have had exposure from more than one building. When a HERTSMI-2 score is less than 11, a CIRS patient can reasonably expect to be safe and not relapse in the building (Shoemaker and Lark 6). But in a study done by Dr. Ritchie Shoemaker and David Lark, the average HERTSMI-2 of residential buildings was found to be 17.6, the average of workplaces 15.5, and the average of schools 17.8 (5-6). So, clearly, exposure to environments that do not meet treatment standards is inevitable if one isn't aware and cautious.

By the time I was diagnosed, I was too sick to go anywhere anyway. I was still living at home, had graduated from high school, and had stopped going to dance and college, so I didn't have an office or school environment to also contend with. But, as a CIRS patient, you must make sure you are living in a safe place, and you must also know the conditions of all of the buildings you spend time in regularly, ideally by testing them, and make sure they will not make you sick. Usually, this includes your living environment and workplace or school.

For your school or workplace, you will likely have no control over the environment. You have to either find a way to work with those in charge or quit. If your living environment is too high in toxins to be safe for you, you can remediate the environment or move somewhere safe. This is where it gets really messy.

If you decide to remediate either your home or office, you must find someone who can remediate it properly to make it a safe environment. You should be able to go to your regular indoor environmental professional (IEP) or mold inspector and remediator, right? Wrong. Right now, the average IEP, mold inspector, and remediator have no idea how to properly assess and remediate at an adequate level for those with CIRS. Most only work at the level that affects people with asthma, allergies, or no health issues, and they are "not aware of the limitations of their testing modalities and will tell their clients their home is 'safe' when they have only done a fairly insensitive test that found nothing" (McMahon). Larry Schwartz, an IEP trained to work with CIRS patients, describes the situation as working under two different paradigms. The majority of IEPs and remediators are trained to assess and remediate within the "traditional paradigm", at the level of spores, but not within the "inflammatory paradigm", at the level of mycotoxins, microbial VOCs, endotoxins, etc. which is what affects those with CIRS (Schwartz).

So what now? Who do you go to? Where do you turn for help? In the absence of an organization that exists to help you know where to go next, you can go to your doctor and ask them for a recommendation, but sadly they may not be able to give one. Doctors in this field are desperate for educated IEPs and remediators, and most do not have one they can refer patients to (Dooley). There are only a handful of IEPs and remediators who are considered qualified and widely trusted by the CIRS medical community to help CIRS patients. Unless they have experience with the CIRS community, how can they be qualified, when there is no widely accepted and accessible continuing education program or certification in place to give them those skills? You can see how this is problematic.

So, after spending likely over a thousand dollars just to get in to see a doctor, get diagnostic lab tests, and test your home, you must now spend potentially thousands more to get your home properly assessed and remediated. If you can't access the qualified professionals capable of proper assessment and remediation, you could go to the cheaper competition who has no idea what they are doing when it comes to CIRS and let them do their thing. But then you'd be paying for essentially nothing, because they have neither the skills nor the tools to remediate your building in a way that will remove the particles that are making you sick.

So, if you can't afford or access the qualified professionals, currently your only option is to fully educate yourself on the subject of remediation when it comes to biotoxins and CIRS – a subject that is still undergoing rigorous study by the professionals in the industry because the "knowledge is constantly expanding" (Dooley). Then, hire a regular, cheaper IEP and remediator, and try to teach them and tell them what to do. And remember, during this time you may be dealing with severe cognitive issues and incapacitating fatigue from CIRS. So you will have to learn all of this complex information and then pay to teach someone how to do their job at an adequate level for your condition, which has made you cognitively and physically disabled.

Okay. Remediation is just too problematic, so you decide to move. Now, you must understand which possessions you can safely clean and bring with you when you move, and which ones will carry those very components that make you sick, making your new environment unsafe. Where do you turn for guidance on this? Well, ideally you would turn to an indoor environmental professional (IEP). But, as we've learned, that isn't really an option unless you can find one trained in CIRS, and afford them. So you must again, with cognitive issues and incapacitating fatigue, learn the details yourself, either through your own research or by purchasing one of the few books or courses designed to help patients manage the different parts of treatment.

Once you learn what can be cleaned and how to clean it, you have to actually do it. Depending on your condition and what items you are cleaning, you may be able to do this yourself. However, if you are very sensitive, you may need someone else to do this cleaning for you, as you will be exposed to more inflammagens when cleaning items from an environment that isn't safe for you. Also keep in mind, you are likely still dealing with fatigue and cognitive issues from CIRS. This cleaning process is incredibly energy and time consuming and can be even more so if you have significant anxiety or OCD like I did.

The other half of this is the additional cost of replacing the items that cannot be safely remediated. Mattresses, upholstered furniture, books, rugs, and wooden items are all porous materials that will be saturated with the particles that make you sick, and they cannot be cleaned to the level required.

If you somehow accomplish all this, pray that your environment stays safe. "Current construction leaves room for a lot of issues" (Smith). And "it's overwhelming how most current construction materials and methods are not helping create environmentally safe homes" (Schwartz).

If you are unable to *keep* your environment safe, you're back to where you were before. You must move or somehow remediate the environment and redo the cleaning process on all of your household items. My experience, again, has been a great example of this. We went through everything it took to get out of the poor environment and into a good one; we cleaned what we could and got rid of what we couldn't. When we finally made it, we made sure to be vigilant. We checked under and behind areas like the sinks and any other water-using appliances daily or weekly. We were vigilant about keeping the bathrooms dry. We also had two air purifiers running 24/7.

We did everything in our power to keep our environment safe. Yet we still faced water damage four months after we moved in when our upstairs neighbor's toilet supply line leaked. Though we were lucky and the apartment management was willing to do things right and bring in a remediation company the very next morning, the process was still daunting, complex, and difficult, as we still had to educate the remediator so he could remediate at the necessary level.

The complexity, the cost, the lack of support, the lack of acknowledgment and acceptance – all these factors are why "hundreds, maybe thousands," of patients are living in tents, in their cars, or quite literally any place they can find just to be able to survive (McMahon). Exposure to the inflammagens has to stop. As one doctor put it, it's like lead or mercury exposure, just a different toxin. "You have to quit putting the toxin in the body if you're going to get well" (Johnson). And, like lead and mercury poisoning, without any intervention, this inflammatory condition can prove deadly (Beshara). It won't say CIRS on the death certificate. But, for some, CIRS is what made the body vulnerable to more acute and fatal illnesses. People are dying from this. Some are stuck working or living in environments that make them sick because they can't afford to even begin treatment. Some, after being given false hope by so many doctors, are not willing to try yet another thing, especially when it would cost them so much. Some have been diagnosed with something else that "no one" understands why they got it. And others are told it's all in their head.

So, for some, this is a slow and agonizing death. It's an avoidable death, but only if you can catch it and somehow afford to treat it.

The reality is, without my family, I would not have gotten better. I would have been slowly declining from where I was in 2018. I wouldn't have been able to hold down a job. I'd have ended up on disability... if I could even get it. Eventually, I might have contracted an acute illness that would result in my death. Or, with my mental health so strongly affected by inflammation and despair, maybe I would have decided it wasn't worth going on. Every day would have been a struggle, every second filled with pain and despair, and no escape. This alternate reality that I escaped, is some people's reality. This has got to change.

Chapter 12
Help and Hope

So what can we do to change this? What more can we do to get people the help they need and keep them from avoidable suffering and death?

After study, research, and interviews with over a dozen experts in the field, I've determined where to begin focusing *my* efforts to make the biggest impact I can and help the most people I can. All of my investigations keep pointing me back to two things: *raising awareness* and *educating the experts*. Pursuing these two outcomes will help, and in some cases solve, many of the difficulties people with environmentally acquired illness (EAI), like CIRS, face. But no one person or organization can do this alone; it must be a "community working together to solve a problem" (DiTulio).

When it comes to educating experts, there is a deficit in nearly every area. Some EAI, like asthma and allergies, are understood by the mainstream and have been treated by practitioners for decades. However, when it comes to EAI like CIRS, from what I have seen in the US, there are only a handful of doctors per state who are capable of recognizing and treating it. Still, much has been accomplished since it was first discovered via the 1997 *Pfiesteria* outbreak at Chesapeake Bay. All the work done since is the very reason I was able to find a doctor who could help me. There is a certification process, created by Dr. Shoemaker and his team, for practitioners to become educated and qualified to treat CIRS. There is an organization, ISEAI, that helps to educate and bring professionals into the fold of EAI knowledge and treatment. Some universities like The University of Arizona (UArizona) offer courses to help educate doctors and other medical personnel on EAI (Reynolds). So there is a lot that has been done, and is being done, to help practitioners become capable of recognizing and treating CIRS. But, as demonstrated by how difficult it is to find a doctor proficient in CIRS diagnosis and treatment, there is still a huge deficit and this effort must continue.[15]

However, there is an even more severe lack of qualified indoor environmental professionals (IEPs) and remediators. This has got to be fixed because every doctor I have spoken with has stated that IEPs and remediators are critical to a patient's full recovery. The doctors themselves need a basic understanding of the concepts of indoor air quality (IAQ) that relate to a patient's recovery so they can educate their patients on the importance of a safe environment. Unfortunately, most do not have the extensive knowledge necessary to teach a patient how to create or find and maintain a safe environment for themselves (Goggin). Even when doctors can provide this help, patients are having to "rely on their own skills" to actually get it done, and many are dealing with cognitive issues, which can greatly contribute to inaccurate test results and other costly mistakes (Smith).

It can't be just any regular inspector. The inspector or the IEP is "diagnosing" the building (DiTulio). If they don't have the knowledge to "diagnose" the building at the depth to which a CIRS patient needs, they simply cannot help the patient. The patient may even tell their inspector/remediator, "My doctor said I need to do this test on my home," but if the inspectors/ remediators don't know what the test is or understand what it does, they might not listen to the patient. "These experts need

---

15   See Appendix A for resources, links to courses, and more information.

to be clear on what they are doing" (Smith) and they need to understand that a more in-depth approach is necessary when dealing with inflammatory illness (DiTulio).

When a sufficiently educated IEP is on board and helping the patient, things are easier on both the patient and the doctor (Goggin). The doctor has an accurate assessment of the state of a patient's living environment, can proceed with treatment, and can better help the patient with this knowledge in hand. And the patient isn't having to be the "expert", and deal with costly mistakes stemming from their physical limitations, cognitive issues, or lack of knowledge on the complexity of indoor environments. So IEPs who are educated to the level necessary for these patients are not only a "wealth of information", but are also critical to getting through the most difficult part of treatment (Johnson).

But, unfortunately, such IEPs are extremely rare. As mentioned in Chapter 11, the majority of IEPs, mold inspectors, and remediators are trained to remediate and assess at the level of spores, the "traditional paradigm", which tends to affect those with asthma, allergies, or no health issues (Schwartz). It's great that they can remediate at this level, but there are two issues with them being able to work *only* at this level. One, there is "scientific evidence indicating that current post-remediation standards are failing persons with CIRS-WDB, persons whose special health needs require a more aggressive post-remediation standard for establishing safe conditions for habitation after water damage" (Schwartz et al. 21). Two, only 5-10% of the population is affected by the "traditional paradigm", whereas 24%, and likely more, of the population has the genetic potential to develop and be affected by CIRS from water-damaged buildings (Schwartz). So the majority of IEPs and remediators are trained to remediate at a level for something that only affects 5-10% of the population, but not at the level that potentially affects 24% or more of the population.

So why are they not trained to assess and remediate further? Well, maybe the biggest contributor to this deficit is that there is no formal and widely available training that IEPs and remediators can take to gain this deeper knowledge and become qualified to help CIRS patients. Those who are qualified are doing what they can to educate others by creating courses or by taking on interested IEPs and contractors and training them in "medically sound remediation."[16] But, beyond this, there isn't much at all that's available in the US. And, because of this lack of educational programs, there is a lack of these qualified experts.

As a result, these experts are in such demand that they can barely keep up with it. In one interview, Larry Schwartz shared how he is passionate to help these people but is so overwhelmed by demand. "We get calls and questions; people that are hurting need help... Everything's urgent. Weekends have no meaning. We do our best to channel them to come through normal hours but our work and catching up on reports and everything – I spend most of my weekends just doing catch-up work. So, yeah, we definitely need help" (Schwartz).

This is why CIRS-proficient IEPs and indoor air quality (IAQ) experts Michael Schrantz and Larry Schwartz, Kelly Reynolds and others in the Zuckerman College of Public Health at the University of Arizona (UArizona), members of the International Society for Environmentally Acquired Illness (ISEAI), members of the American Council for Accredited Certification (ACAC), along with other organizations and individuals in this field, are all working together to create a credible, well-rounded,

---

16 Medically sound remediation is a term used by professionals to refer to assessment and remediation that safeguards the health of individuals affected by indoor air quality. If you are an IEP, remediator, or professional in the building/indoor environment field and are interested in learning from one of these qualified professionals, you can inquire about Larry Schwartz's training at www.safestartiaq.com/contact-us/ or call (708) 663-2073.

and far-reaching continuing education process for IEPs and remediators that would be available globally.[17]

Another group of experts necessary to helping people with CIRS, who are lacking in available education on the subject, are those experts involved in the construction of buildings and homes. It's "not only the type of materials used in construction, but even various construction methods" that contribute to buildings' vulnerability to water damage, biotoxins, and formaldehyde and VOCs that off-gas from building materials (Schwartz). Larry Schwartz says, "There are better materials and... better structural materials that are less likely to have mold on them coming in or to develop mold", but "building standards are much more general; they leave a lot of decisions up to the contractor.... Most of the construction standards go more into the functional use of things. They don't generally specify specific building materials... I don't know of any communities that have what I would call environmental construction standards." This lack of standards allows for these issues to be ignored despite the fact that "indoor air pollution is probably the most influential factor when it comes to health overall" (Smith).

---

17 Though much of this certification is still under development, it is intended to be a "graduate certificate in Environmentally Acquired Illnesses (EAI) [and] will provide additional training to professionals already in the field" (Reynolds). The courses will include an introduction to EAI, education on quality assessment of indoor environments, "Quantitative Human Health Risk Assessment", and a customizable section to help set up professionals so they can apply this knowledge in their areas of interest (e.g. remediation, consulting builders on building CIRS-safe homes, public health, etc.). To ensure that the information that makes up the courses stays up to date, the program will be flexible and continuously updated (Reynolds). Though the certification itself is still under development, some of the courses that will make up the certification are currently being offered at the University of Arizona (UArizona). To support this certification project via donations or in-kind contributions contact: reynolds@arizona.edu.

Because this has gone on for so long and so many buildings are built without such standards, "doctors are seeing more and more of this unique sensitivity in the patient population" (Goggin). Buildings constructed to maintain good indoor air quality are key to keeping so many people safe and healthy. Newer, more mold- and toxin-impervious buildings need to be built. To have the research and projects to do so and to eventually raise building standards, we need architects, builders, contractors, IEPs, and other experts who are up to date on the latest research and knowledge. To have such experts, we need well-rounded and credible educational programs like certifications and continuing education units (CEU).

But these adequately educated experts that we are trying to increase by educational programs are themselves critical to *creating* these educational programs. And, as I've said before, IEPs, medical experts, architects, and other professionals who have the necessary knowledge are few and far between. For example, the two IEPs – Larry Schwartz and Michael Schrantz – currently working on the University of Arizona (UArizona) certification process are taking on this project despite being overwhelmed with clients and projects that demand the expertise that few like them possess. And up to this point, they've been *donating* their time. Though many are moved to action and will donate as much time as they are able, the fact is "these people are in such high demand that they must be paid for their time. These are the people who can make the most difference, and we need funding to get them together and working towards these goals" (Schrantz).

≡

To get this much-needed funding and to further progress, we need to continue efforts to raise public awareness and support for CIRS. This is where I have found a place in advocacy for this condition. Though I do not have funding of my own to give, I have my story to tell. I've shared my experiences and my pain. I've shared what I've learned from research and talking to experts who work with CIRS patients every day, who see them struggle to overcome impossible odds and obstacles. My experiences and learning all of this has moved me to action. I've come to realize that I can be a voice for those with CIRS and that I can help raise awareness and support for CIRS patients, starting with this book.

And for such a complex condition in such need of support and awareness, to which approximately a *quarter* of the population is susceptible to contracting, there is so much more that needs to be done. For example, we need to have more projects and programs for educating professionals, and these programs need funding. If these programs are unable to easily and efficiently accept donations themselves, we need organizations that can do so on their behalf. Once these professionals are educated and qualified to help, we need networks and organizations that are able to help CIRS patients easily find and access this information free of charge. We need to find ways to make these professionals not only easy to find, but also easy for a CIRS patient to afford.

If you want to help achieve these goals, there are a few things you can do. First, reading this book is a huge help in and of itself because it raises *your* awareness. So if you've gotten this far, thank you. Second, you can share what you've learned. Tell people, start a conversation about indoor air quality (IAQ) and its impact on people's health. Tell people about this book, or about the fact that people are experiencing medically-induced homelessness and living in tents or out of their car. Lastly, you can keep up to date on the newest projects and information. The Surviving Mold website, survivingmold.com, and ISEAI's website, iseai.org, are great places to keep up with the latest information and research in the CIRS/EAI field. You can also follow me as I continue my journey. This is just the beginning of the advocacy work I'll be doing for CIRS. You can follow me on social media[18] where I'll be sharing my journey as well as information on advocacy projects.

I will continue to be a voice for the silent quarter – for all those whose lives are being affected or destroyed by CIRS, for all those who have had their voices taken from them by this incapacitating condition – and I look forward with hope as we progress down this road together.

**See Appendix A for resources on CIRS
and EAI doctors, IEPs, and more.**

---

18   **Instagram:** vivianel89 **Facebook:** www.facebook.com/viviane.lovato.37/
LinkedIn: www.linkedin.com/in/vivianelovato

References

Beshara, Mary. Interview. Conducted by Viviane Lovato, 27 June 2020.

DiTulio, Margaret. Interview. Conducted by Viviane Lovato, 19 June 2020.

Dooley, M. and McMahon, S. "A Comprehensive Review of Mold Research Literature from 2011 - 2018." *Internal Medicine Review*, 2020. *Crossref*, doi:10.18103/imr.v6i1.836.

Dooley, Ming. Interview. Conducted by Viviane Lovato, 24 Aug 2020.

Goggin, Linda. Interview. Conducted by Viviane Lovato, 3 July 2020.

Gupta, Sandeep. Interview. Conducted by Viviane Lovato, 30 July 2020.

Johnson, Karen. Interview. Conducted by Viviane Lovato, June 2020.

"Lab Tests." *Surviving Mold*, www.survivingmold.com/diagnosis/lab-tests. Accessed 8 Sept. 2020.

McMahon, Scott. Interview. Conducted by Viviane Lovato, 18 July and 25 Aug 2020.

Reynolds, Kelly. Interview. Conducted by Viviane Lovato, 15 July and 14 Sept 2020.

Schrantz, Michael. Interview. Conducted by Viviane Lovato, May 2020.

Schwartz, L., Weatherman, G., Schrantz, M., Spates, W., Charlton, J., Berndtson, K. and Shoemaker, R. "Indoor Environmental Professionals Panel of Surviving Mold Consensus Statement." *Surviving Mold*, 2016, www.survivingmold.com/shoemaker-protocol/community/indoor-environmental-professionals-panel-of-surviving-mold-consensus-statement.

Schwartz, Larry. Interview. Conducted by Viviane Lovato, 4 June and 26 Aug 2020.

Shoemaker, R., Johnson, K., Jim, L., Berry, Y., Dooley, M., Ryan, J. and McMahon, S. "Diagnostic Process for Chronic Inflammatory Response Syndrome (CIRS): A Consensus Statement Report of the Consensus Committee of Surviving Mold." *Internal Medicine Review*, vol. 4, no. 5, 2018, www.survivingmold.com/MEDICAL_CONSENSUS_STATEMENT_10_30_15.PDF.

Shoemaker, R. C. and Lark, D. "HERTSMI-2 and ERMI: Correlating Human Health Risk with Mold Specific QPCR in Water-Damaged Buildings." *Surviving Mold*, 2016, www.survivingmold.com/Publications/HERTSMI-2_AND_ERMI_5_22_2016__CORRELATING_HUMAN_HEALTH_RISK_WITH_MOLD_SPECIFIC_QPCR_IN_WATER_DAMAGED_BUILD-INGS_CLEAN.pdf.

Smith, Jennifer. Interview. Conducted by Viviane Lovato, 15 June 2020.

Appendix A

Resources

Information on CIRS

CIRS diagnostic process consensus statement:
internalmedicinereview.org/index.php/imr/article/view/718

Course – Mold Illness Made Simple (MIMS):
This is the course I refer to in Chapter 11, and I think it is a great resource for patients, patients' relatives, professionals who are curious about CIRS, and anyone else looking to gain a basic understanding of the complex illness CIRS and how it is treated.

To find more information or to purchase the course go to:
www.moldillnessmadesimple.com?aff=vivianelovato
(If you use this link/URL to purchase the course, I will receive a portion as an affiliate marketer)

Websites

Surviving Mold:
survivingmold.com

CIRS certified and CIRS proficient doctors and practitioners:
www.survivingmold.com/shoemaker-protocol/
Certified-Physicians-Shoemaker-Protocol

www.survivingmold.com/shoemaker-protocol/
surviving-mold-proficiency-partners-diplomates

Information on getting certified and trained to treat CIRS:
www.survivingmold.com/store1/shoemaker-protocol-module

Indoor Environmental Professionals Panel of Surviving Mold
Consensus Statement: www.survivingmold.com/shoemaker-
protocol/community/indoor-environmental-professionals-panel-
of-surviving-mold-consensus-statement
(At the time this book was written, an updated consensus statement
was in the works. When published, this updated version should be
available at survivingmold.com.)

ISEAI:
iseai.org

Clinician and IEP list:
iseai.org/find-a-professional/

Education:
iseai.org/education/

The Institute for Functional Medicine:
ifm.org

Directory of Functional Medicine doctors:
(Not all Functional Medicine doctors are CIRS proficient)
www.ifm.org/find-a-practitioner/

ERMI, HERTSMI-2, and Other Environmental Testing:

EnviroBiomics, Inc – www.envirobiomics.com
Mycometrics – www.mycometrics.com

VCS Testing

Surviving Mold – www.survivingmold.com/diagnosis/
visual-contrast-sensitivity-vcs
VCSTest.com – www.vcstest.com

Appendix B

Has CIRS Been "Proven"?

This is a topic I am quite reluctant to speak on. I feel it is important that we talk about this, but who am I to speak on it? I am not a doctor, I am not an IEP, and I'm no expert. I'm nobody. But I have lived it, I've researched it, and I've talked to many of the experts. So I will share with you what I've learned, and you can decide for yourself, just as I have.

Throughout this book, I've walked you through my experience of living with CIRS. I've shared the experience of finding a doctor, getting diagnosed, and seeing the incredible impact of treatment. I talked to you about the loved ones I've watched go through the same thing, and I've talked to you about the stories I've heard from doctors about their patients' experiences, as well as all the scientific work they have done on the subject. This all gives me a certain intimate knowledge of this biotoxin-induced illness, and I've tried to give you that same knowledge through this book.

So let's start with the question: What does it take for something to "be proven" in scientific and medical terms? For science, proof comes from using the process of the Scientific Method: observations lead to a hypothesis, this hypothesis leads to predictions, which are then tested by experiments and studies. "If your predictions come true, your hypothesis becomes a theory" (McMahon). As "research is repeated by others, validating original findings" (Dooley), "the theory becomes accepted by the mainstream" (McMahon). Different professionals have different opinions on when exactly in this process something is "proven", so "it is unclear at what point in this process one considers something 'proven'" (McMahon).

Additionally, the deeper I went into my research the more complex it got. CIRS is complex in and of itself. Not only do the health effects of this illness affect several systems in the body, making it complicated in that manner, but *how* it triggers these health effects is even more complicated. "There are 30 different classes of things that can trigger the innate immune system" (McMahon) which are found in water-damaged buildings. There are endotoxins, nano-sized particulates, microbial VOCs, building material VOCs, etc. (Schwartz et al. 4). And, even if we simplify it down to just the mold, there are different emissions and components of mold that can contribute to the illness, like mycotoxins and microbial VOCs, whose impact greatly depends on the environment in which, and on which, the mold is growing.

All of this makes CIRS incredibly complex to study and evaluate. Nevertheless, it has been done successfully, and the results have been validated. Dr. McMahon, in the last several years, has been following up and validating over 20 years of CIRS-specific research by Dr. Shoemaker (McMahon). And in a study done by Dr. Ming Dooley and Dr. Scott McMahon in January 2020, they looked at existing medical literature from 2011-2018 to determine whether current literature supports adverse health effects caused by exposure to mold and water-damaged buildings. They concluded that "current literature supports multi-system adverse human health effects in those chronically exposed to indoor microbial growth/dampness" (Dooley and McMahon 2). Tying this back to the Scientific Method, Dr. McMahon stated in an interview that the literature "shows the phenomenon, [and] CIRS is the explanation or hypothesis of how and why."

So what about those articles that clearly dismiss the health effects of microbial growth and water-damaged buildings, and say things like "Despite a voluminous literature on the subject, the causal association remains weak and unproven, particularly with respect to causation by mycotoxins" (Hardin et al.)? Well, under further scrutiny, many of the works that claim such things have been shown to have hidden biases, conflicts of interest, errors, or are based upon assumptions made in other works that have already been disproven.

An example of such can be found in the article "Adverse human health effects associated with molds in the indoor environment" from the American College of Occupational and Environmental Medicine (ACOEM), quoted above. It's been shown that this article's "author selection, development, peer review, and publication…. involved a series of seemingly biased and ethically dubious decisions and ad hoc methods" (Craner). Authors of this article were "professional mold defense expert witnesses" – experts who testify on behalf of multi-billion dollar companies, typically in encounters where an individual has lost their health, home, job, savings, even family, and is going up against a corporate giant or legal team to try to get enough to get whole and start over – and these authors were not upfront about this conflict of interest (McMahon). Not only that, but it also "omitted or inadequately acknowledged research validating the association between mold and building-related symptoms" (Craner). For example, it's much more than just mycotoxins that make people sick. As Dr. McMahon stated and Dr. Ming Dooley reiterated, "mycotoxins are a tiny percent… of what affects people" (Dooley). With a closer look at the mathematics and "using the Scientific Method, one can easily see that the premise of the 2002 ACOEM article is false" (McMahon).

These kinds of issues can be found in several publications that dismiss mold's effects on the immune system and inflammation. Some are based on this very ACOEM article, relying on it to support a similar conclusion. Others have strong and clear biases. In one such article, the bias was so clear that one of the authors "considered removing his name from the paper" (Armstrong 5).

So where do the "powers that be" stand on this? In a recent review, the World Health Organization (WHO) concludes that "the most important effects are increased prevalences of respiratory symptoms, allergies and asthma as well as perturbation of the immunological system" (WHO). "Perturbation" or disturbance of the immunological system describes what CIRS does because it essentially revs up the innate immune system and causes chronic and systemic inflammation.

The National Institute of Environmental Health Sciences (NIEHS) states that "symptoms stemming from mold spore exposure may include: nasal and sinus congestion, eye irritation, blurred vision, sore throat, chronic cough, and skin rash" (NIEHS), not mentioning anything about the effects of mold, or its byproducts, on the immune system. The Centers for Disease Control and Prevention's (CDC) stance is that "mold can cause a stuffy nose, sore throat, coughing or wheezing, burning eyes, or skin rash" (CDC), again not mentioning anything about the immune system. And the National Institute of Occupational Safety and Health (NIOSH) only mentions allergies, hypersensitivity pneumonitis, and asthma when it talks of the health effects of mold (NIOSH). However, in 2012, NIOSH evaluated the health effects of exposure to water damaged buildings and whether a Visual Contrast Sensitivity (VCS) test is a reliable indicator of whether someone is having adverse health effects from a water-damaged building (Thomas et al.). The people in the water damaged building "had higher prevalences of... rashes and nasal, lower respiratory, and constitutional symptoms" than those in the building without water damage, and the VCS scores of those in the water damaged environment were indeed lower than those in the environment that was not water damaged (Thomas et al.). So what exactly are "constitutional symptoms"? Well, they encompass generalized symptoms such as fatigue, chronic pain, and headache, all of which are associated with CIRS.

So, though some of the larger organizations imply or outright state that this is not an issue, mold's effects on the immune system seem to be supported by the majority of literature on the subject. So why aren't its effects on the immune system widely accepted and acknowledged, and why is it still so disputed?

The truth is, even when multitudes of studies are done and published in all the right places, "it might not be accepted if it's too different or too new" (Gupta). Others closely involved in discussions on mold and its health effects point to the fact that "trillions of dollars are at stake" in this issue, and insurance companies and entities that have previously dismissed mold's health effects stand to lose millions (McMahon). Still others say that it will take time and that the up-and-coming professionals need to be taught about it (Goggin). Dr. McMahon, referring to the knowledge gap that seems to exist between doctors from his age bracket and the upcoming, says, "We simply were not taught enough in med school because the information wasn't there. Newer providers have a much better understanding of immune system concepts and readily understand CIRS."

Regardless of exactly how or why, different factors build on one another to create a barrier to progress and acceptance for CIRS. But there are still many things we can do to break down this barrier. More research and studies will help. Dr. McMahon says, "I think we have moved on to the theory stage and will move into the accepted-by-everybody stage as universities and other non-CIRS researchers look at CIRS and reproduce the work Dr. Shoemaker and I have published." Discussing and raising awareness for CIRS and EAI does and will help as well. Educating our experts, our doctors, our IEPs, our builders and architects, as well as making sure there is standardized teaching that professionals can be confident in and even get a certification from, is yet another thing that is being worked on and can be done to progress things for CIRS patients.

From what I've experienced and from what I've learned from the experts and the scientific/medical research, mold's effect on the immune system is very real and very dangerous. But it seems that there are those who are determined to ignore an immense amount of research and say that mold's effects on the immune system are a myth, there are those who say there is simply not enough research for them to consider it "proven", and there are those who say that CIRS is very real and more research is critical to furthering acknowledgment and acceptance.

Regardless, I've lived this. I've seen the effects of these inflammagens and the effects of removal from exposure and treatment firsthand. So I hope that professionals continue to dig deeper into this issue with research, and that we continue to raise awareness. I hope that soon we can all stop debating *if* mold affects people's health via the immune system and inflammation, and focus our time and energy on helping people.

References for Appendix B

Armstrong, D. "Amid Suits Over Mold, Experts Wear Two Hats: Authors of Science Paper Often Cited by Defense Also Help in Litigation." *Wall Street Journal*, 2007,www.armstrongjournal-ism.com/wp-content/uploads/2014/12/Amid-Suits-Over-Mold-Experts-Wear-Two-Hats.pdf.

Craner, J. Abstract of "A Critique of the ACOEM Statement on Mold: Undisclosed Conflicts of Interest in the Creation of an 'Evidence-Based' Statement." *International Journal of Occupational and Environmental Health*, vol. 14, no. 4, 2008, pp. 283–98. *Crossref*, doi:10.1179/oeh.2008.14.4.283.

Dooley, M. and McMahon, S. "A Comprehensive Review of Mold Research Literature from 2011 - 2018." *Internal Medicine Review*, 2020. *Crossref*, doi:10.18103/imr.v6i1.836.

Dooley, Ming. Interview. Conducted by Viviane Lovato, 24 Aug 2020.

Goggin, Linda. Interview. Conducted by Viviane Lovato, 3 July 2020.

Gupta, Sandeep. Interview. Conducted by Viviane Lovato, 30 July 2020.

Hardin, B.D., Kelman, B. J. and Saxon, A. Abstract of "Adverse Human Health Effects Associated with Molds in the Indoor Environment." *Journal of Occupational and Environmental*

Medicine, vol. 45, no. 5, 2003, pp. 470–78. *Crossref*, doi:10.1097/00043764-200305000-00006.

McMahon, Scott. Interview. Conducted by Viviane Lovato, 18 July and 25 Aug 2020.

"Mold | CDC." *Centers for Disease Control and Prevention*, www.cdc.gov/mold/default.htm. Accessed 23 July 2020.

"Mold." *National Institute of Environmental Health Sciences*, www.niehs.nih.gov/health/topics/agents/mold/index.cfm. Accessed 23 July 2020.

National Institute of Occupational Safety and Health. "CDC - Indoor Environmental Quality: Dampness and Mold in Buildings - NIOSH Workplace Safety and Health Topic." *Centers for Disease Control and Prevention*, www.cdc.gov/niosh/topics/indoorenv/mold.html. Accessed 23 July 2020.

Schwartz, L., Weatherman, G., Schrantz, M., Spates, W., Charlton, J., Berndtson, K. and Shoemaker, R. "Indoor Environmental Professionals Panel of Surviving Mold Consensus Statement." *Surviving Mold*, www.survivingmold.com/shoemaker-protocol/community/indoor-environmental-professionals-panel-of-surviving-mold-consensus-statement. Accessed 7 July 2020.

Thomas, G., Burton N.C., Mueller C., Page E. and Vesper S. Abstract of "Comparison of Work-Related Symptoms and Visual Contrast Sensitivity between Employees at a Severely Water-Damaged School and a School without Significant Water Damage." *American Journal of Industrial Medicine*, vol. 55, no. 9, 2012, pp. 844–54. *Crossref*, doi:10.1002/ajim.22059.

World Health Organization. "WHO Guidelines for Indoor Air Quality: Dampness and Mould." *World Health Organization*, 17 June 2020, www.who.int/airpollution/guidelines/dampness-mould/en.